VIRUS DISEASES
A Layman's Handbook

Also by David Locke

ENZYMES—THE AGENTS OF LIFE

VIRUSES: THE SMALLEST ENEMY

VIRUS DISEASES
A Layman's Handbook

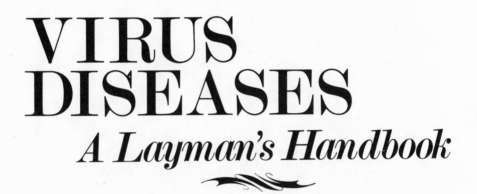

David Locke

CROWN PUBLISHERS, INC., NEW YORK

Printed in the United States of America
Published simultaneously in Canada
by General Publishing Company Limited

Library of Congress Cataloging in Publication Data

Locke, David Millard, 1929-
   Virus diseases—a layman's handbook.

   Bibliography: p.
   1. Virus diseases. I. Title.
RC114.5.L57   616.9'51   77-20115
ISBN 0-517-53279-4

Designed by RUTH KOLBERT SMERECHNIAK

Contents

Systematic Table of Contents*

*Rubrics that correspond to article titles are printed in capital letters; those that serve only to group articles together are printed in capital and small letters. Many entries logically belong in more than one category. In each such case a "main" location is somewhat arbitrarily selected, where the rubric appears as it normally would; at "secondary" locations the rubric appears also, but in parentheses.

Prefatory Note

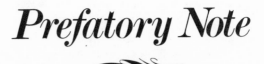

THIS BOOK and HOW TO USE IT

This book is about virus diseases in general, but mostly it concerns the individual virus diseases, their symptoms, the course they are likely to follow, and the probable outcome. It lists the signs that help diagnose each disease, indicates the accepted therapies, and gives the expectations of their success.

This book is not intended to be a guide for self-diagnosis and treatment, however. Nor will it serve as a substitute for consulting a physician. (The man who acts as his own physician—like the one who acts as his own lawyer—has a fool for a client.) But it may help in deciding when consulting a physician is necessary and when it is not.

The purpose of the book is to inform, to tell the reader the things that today's harried physician rarely has time to tell him. The day of the family doctor, who patiently explained what was wrong, what he was doing, and what we might expect, is long gone. The average person today does not even have a family doctor; he encounters a busy, even over-worked, member of a medical team in a hospital emergency room or at a medical clinic. And he gets little in the way of information—only an incomprehensible list of tests to be performed, and a prescription.

Not only do we not get to talk to our doctors anymore; they find it increasingly hard to tell us what's wrong if we do. Modern medicine is becoming increasingly specialized, and the modern physician is becoming less and less able to converse outside the jargon of his specialty. "It's too complicated," we are told when we press. "You wouldn't understand."

This book is dedicated to the proposition that virus diseases are not too complicated, and that you will understand them. It attempts to lay out clearly and simply what it means to have any particular virus disease—what is happening and what you can expect to happen.

Now a word on how to use the book. It can, of course, be read through—if the reader is interested in learning about all the different virus diseases and how they relate to one another. To facilitate such a course, a Systematic Table of Contents is provided, which, when followed, will permit the reader to approach the diseases in a logical order.

But this volume is also designed to be a reference book for the reader who wants to learn what there is to know about a single virus disease, one that he has himself perhaps, or a friend or relative has, or simply a disease that he has read or heard about. For such use, the articles are given in alphabetical order, with numerous cross-references for alternate names. (For example, the rubrics RUBELLA and MEASLES, GERMAN both refer the reader to the article GERMAN MEASLES.) The regular Table of Contents includes a list of the article entries only, so that the reader can consult it initially to determine whether or not an entry appears, and under what rubric.

The index, of course, provides another means of finding entries of interest. Through it, for instance, the reader can learn what diseases are characterized by particular symptoms or are treated with particular remedies.

Within the articles, cross-references—indicated by entry titles in capital letters—refer the reader to related articles. These supplement what he has read or provide information on similar diseases.

Although the number of technical terms in the articles has been kept to a minimum, and most of those that occur are defined explicitly or implicitly in the text, a few—some two dozen—that occur repeatedly in the text are defined in a glossary at the end of the book. (In this way, the constant repetition of a few standard definitions is avoided.) To alert the reader that a word is in the glossary, on its first appearance in an article such a word is given in italics.*

---

*This means that other italicized words must be avoided, a practice that has been adhered to at the expense of some violation of standard usage. Thus, book titles and foreign words are placed within quotation marks, and the official names of organisms, which usually take the form *Escherichia coli,* or as abbreviated, *E. coli,* are printed in regular type.

Wherever possible, article entries cover single diseases, but in the case of a few closely related ailments (such as the Eastern, Western, and Venezuelan equine encephalitises), to avoid the presence of several nearly identical articles, the diseases are covered together (in this case, under the rubric EQUINE ENCEPHALITIS). Most entries deal with single disease entities regardless of how many different viruses cause them. (Thus, THE COMMON COLD may be caused by many different kinds of viruses, but appears as one entry.)

On the other hand, a few articles (such as COXSACKIE OR ECHO VIRUS INFECTION) deal with the various manifestations of infection by one or a few closely related viruses because the disorders they cause are quite varied and not recognized as discrete diseases. Also, in a few instances (such as ENCEPHALITIS), damage to a particular organ system is covered in an article entry even though it may be a manifestation of a number of different diseases, provided that it sometimes occurs as a clearly identified disorder on its own.

In his reading, particularly of older materials, the reader may occasionally encounter references to what are described as virus diseases but which are not covered in this book. The explanation is quite simple. The disease is probably one of a small group—psittacosis, or parrot fever, is the best-known example—caused by a family of organisms once considered to be viruses but now known not to be. These organisms, which are variously known as chlamydiae, bedsoniae, and miygawanellae, multiply only within cells, as viruses do, but they maintain their own identity within the cell and reproduce by division, both properties quite different from those of viruses. (Besides psittacosis, a disease of birds only occasionally transmitted to man, the family includes several truly human diseases: trachoma and inclusion conjunctivitis, both eye ailments, and lymphogranuloma venereum, a little discussed but fairly common venereal disease.)

Another group of disorders, the rickettsial diseases, are sometimes discussed along with virus diseases because rickettsiae, the causative organisms, are also almost wholly dependent on cells for their growth and multiplication. (This group includes typhus and Rocky Mountain spotted fever, which are carried by lice and ticks respectively, and Q fever, a disease of cattle conveyed to man by dusts laden with the organism.) Both the chlamydiae and the rickettsiae are susceptible to the action of ordinary antibiotics, as viruses are not. Hence, the whole mode of treatment of the disorders they cause is quite different from that of the virus diseases, and those diseases are not covered here.

In July and August 1976 an outbreak of a mysterious malady hit participants at an American Legion convention in Philadelphia. In all some 30 people died, out of 180 believed to have been afflicted with what quickly came to be known as Legionnaires' disease. Early attempts to identify the agent responsible for the disease ruled out all known viruses and bacteria, and for a time the illness was thought to be due to a chemical toxin. Ultimately, however, the agent was shown to be a previously unknown bacterium. In retrospective studies the same organism was found to have caused earlier outbreaks of disease, and subsequent minor epidemics also have occurred. Not being a virus, the Legionnaires' disease agent, like the organisms just described, is susceptible to antibiotics, and Legionnaires' disease, too, finds no place in this book.

Finally, any discussion of this book would be incomplete without a word of thanks to a succession of secretaries in the Department of Humanities at the Illinois Institute of Technology, whose patience and diligence helped me to complete the manuscript.

Introduction

~~~~~

VIRUSES and VIRUS DISEASES

The virus diseases are extraordinary in their diversity. Included among them is the most common of all diseases, the cold—responsible for one billion episodes of disease every year in the United States alone, more than the cases of all other diseases combined. Also included is that deadliest of diseases, rabies; with one or two exceptions, everyone who has ever contracted this disease has died of it. And what may be mildest of ailments, warts, for most people, little more than a nuisance. Also, the most contagious of diseases, measles; before the advent of the measles vaccine, more than 97 percent of the world's population managed to catch this disease. And possibly even that most mysterious of maladies, cancer—no one yet knows exactly what causes it, but viruses almost surely play a part.

The only obvious feature that these diseases have in common is, in fact, that they are all caused by viruses. What, then, are viruses, and how do they cause diseases of such diversity?

The viruses consist of tiny particles, minute half-crystalline arrays of protein and *nucleic acid* molecules, so small as to be invisible in ordinary microscopes, but large enough to be readily perceived in the electron microscope. Outside of living cells they are simple inert chemicals; inside them, they spring into life, taking over the cellular machinery and converting the cells into factories for making new virus particles. In doing

1

so, they kill or badly cripple the cells; and when this has happened to enough cells, the body processes are interfered with, and the symptoms of disease appear. Each kind of virus has a propensity to attack a particular type of body cell, and the nature of the cells attacked determines the course of the disease that results. This, in a nutshell, is how viruses act and how they are able to cause such a wide spectrum of diseases, but of course the detailed picture is much more complicated.*

To cause fresh cases of disease, viruses must move from person to person, and they do so in a variety of ways. Many viruses, such as the measles virus, are transmitted via the respiratory tract; that is, virus-laden droplets are emitted into the air by coughing or sneezing, and then someone else breathes them in. Or virus-rich saliva or nasal fluid contaminates utensils or the surroundings, and is passed on to others indirectly; this seems to be mainly how colds spread. Other viruses, such as that of infectious hepatitis, are conveyed from person to person by the fecal-oral route, which is to say that viruses in the feces ultimately find their way onto the hands or utensils and are ingested with food or water. Some viruses pass from one person to another simply by direct contact; this seems to be the case with the warts virus. Still other viruses must be inserted under the skin: with yellow fever and other arbovirus diseases, this is done by a biting insect; with rabies, it is accomplished by the bite of a rabid animal; and with serum hepatitis, the hypodermic of a physician or a narcotics addict can equally well do the job.

Sometimes the spread is very easy—virtually everybody within sight of a measles patient is contaminated, even though the virus is not especially hardy and does not survive long outside the body. Smallpox, too, is incredibly contagious, and this virus is persistent, so much so that special efforts—like the burning of bedclothes—must be resorted to, to decontaminate the sickroom.

But many virus diseases are difficult to transmit, and they spread slowly. Even the common cold does not move around as easily as might be supposed. In a study of couples living together, a cold was spread successfully from one partner to the other in less than 40 percent of the cases.

In their patterns of spread, virus diseases tend to be either *endemic* or *epidemic*. That is to say, either they are around more or less all the time, hitting any new susceptible person who happens to be exposed, or they

---

*For a fuller discussion of viruses and their activities, the reader is invited to consult the author's *Viruses: The Smallest Enemy* (Crown, 1974).

come and go in great waves, sometimes attacking nearly everyone in sight, sometimes all but disappearing completely.

Within the body, viruses follow a number of courses. Some virus infections, like warts, are strictly local. Others, like the common cold, are superficial but cause a degree of general illness. In both such cases, the virus does not move very far in the body, and the damaged cells are all near the portal of entry.

In most virus diseases, however, the course of the infection is roughly as follows: The virus begins to multiply locally in any susceptible cells it encounters, but very quickly it makes its way into the bloodstream, where it invades certain cells and in them is carried to all parts of the body. At this point a generalized feverish illness usually breaks out. And now the virus concentrates its attack on particular tissues or organs and produces the characteristic symptoms of the disease. In mumps, the salivary glands are hit, causing the jaw to swell; in hepatitis, the liver is affected and jaundice results; in measles, German measles, and chicken pox, the skin is the site of attack, and a pox or rash the outcome of it. When essential organs are damaged extensively, as the brain is in rabies, death results.

Most virus diseases are acute; that is, they develop quickly, reach a climax, and either overwhelm the patient's defenses or succumb to them. This is the familiar pattern observed with all the virus diseases referred to above. But there is increasing recognition that some virus diseases follow a different path—more like that of the chronic diseases of old age. These are the so-called slow virus diseases, in which the virus remains in the body for months or years, causing a slow and irregular deterioration. Although the list of diseases known to be in this category is small, and includes such little-known disorders as systemic lupus erythematosus, it is growing. And authorities are beginning to suspect that more and more of the degenerative diseases, such as multiple sclerosis and arthritis, belong on this list.

Cancer is a rather special case of its own. In some respects it seems to resemble the slow virus diseases, but the chief hallmark of cancer is not degeneration but proliferation. What causes cancer cells to proliferate out of control is still not known, but it is clear that one factor that can start the process off is virus infection. We know that viruses cause cancer in animals, and there is increasing evidence that they are involved in some forms of human cancer. Even if viruses are implicated in cancer, however, they do not cause cancer in the same way that they cause other diseases. What they would have to do in cancer is alter the normal cells of the body, transform them into cancer cells, and it is these transformed cells that would develop into full-fledged cancer.

In their various attacks on the body, viruses encounter a number of obstacles, some simple passive barriers to their advance, others active defenses thrown up deliberately by the body. The passive barriers consist of such things as the hard outer layer of the skin and the liquid secretions of the nose and throat. Among the active defenses are (1) the protein *antibodies* in the blood, which selectively attach themselves to the virus particles and render those particles incapable of invading cells; (2) certain highly active cells in the blood that engulf the virus particles and digest them; and (3) *interferon,* a substance that is released by virus-infected cells and conveys a degree of virus resistance to other cells in the neighborhood.

Taken together, these defenses are quite effective in dispatching most virus infections. But they are far from perfect, and man has developed ways of enhancing their action; this forms the basis of most antivirus control measures. To begin with, it is possible to isolate antibodies from blood samples, drawn from many persons, in the form of *gamma globulin,* and give it to others to supplement their own antibodies. Gamma globulin taken from persons recovering from a virus disease, and known as *immune globulin,* is especially effective against the particular virus involved.

Because gamma globulins, being foreign proteins, are quite easily destroyed in the body, they are not very effective virus fighters. Much better results are obtained with vaccines. Composed of *killed* or weakened *viruses,* these stimulate the host to produce his own antibodies, just as a natural infection would, but they do not produce the symptoms of disease.

Recently, scientists have begun to explore ways of stimulating the body's immunity system, which operates in part through antibodies, to render it more active in general. One way of doing this is with a tuberculosis vaccine, named BCG, which seems to help fight cancer of various kinds. Also, several new drugs are thought to act as immunotherapeutic agents, as substances of this type are called. One such drug, levamisole, is active against herpes and influenza viruses and against certain cancers; another, inosiplex, is also reported to be effective against herpes virus and against the rhinoviruses, which cause colds; a third, isoprinosine, has been tested successfully against rhinoviruses, as well as herpes, hepatitis, influenza, and smallpox viruses.

Finally, researchers are looking at means for taking better advantage of interferon in the fight against viruses. Purified interferon obtained from cells of human origin has been shown to be a useful antivirus substance when given soon after exposure, but because it is produced in cells in minute amounts, interferon is very hard to come by. Someday scientists may find ways to make interferon in the laboratory or to obtain it from especially *cultured* cells, but in the meantime they are looking for materials that will cause the body to step up its own production of interferon. A number of such "interferon-inducers" are being actively studied. One, called poly I:C, has been quite effective in animal tests, but less so in tests with human beings. Nonetheless, there is real hope that an effective interferon-inducer for human use will soon be discovered.

Besides their work on beefing up man's natural defenses against viruses, scientists have also been searching for drugs that are themselves directly active against viruses. The search has not been easy because, since viruses function only within cells, it is difficult to halt their action without harming the body cells. Nevertheless, scientists have discovered a number of drugs that are already finding some limited use against virus diseases. One such drug is methisazone, which is active only against the smallpox virus. With the virtual elimination of smallpox from the world, the future for methisazone looks bleak.

Another drug that has found limited use against viruses is idoxuridine. This substance is active against the herpes, or cold-sore virus, but since it is quite toxic, it is limited to the special case of herpes infections in the eye, where the drug need not enter the general circulation. Also, there is a drug called amantadine that prevents influenza. It is not widely used, partly because the FDA has insisted that it undergo extensive testing in human beings against each new strain of the flu virus that appears.

Besides these drugs that have already found some application against virus diseases, a number of others are waiting in the wings, having undergone various levels of testing—in some parts of the world where requirements are less stringent than they are in the United States, several of the drugs are already in use. Among the many drugs in this category are ribavirin, vidarabine, and phosphonoacetic acid, all of which are active against herpes viruses, with ribavirin also effective against hepatitis and influenza viruses. These drugs are not without drawbacks, however; both ribavirin and vidarabine, for instance, are reported to cause birth defects in experimental animals when given to females during pregnancy. But, again, there is hope. So many substances are showing activity against viruses in tests that researchers are growing more confident some will prove to be useful drugs.

Yet, today—as it has been since the 18th century, when Edward Jenner discovered how to prevent smallpox—the main way of controlling virus diseases remains . . . vaccination. In fact, smallpox is the best testimony to the effectiveness of vaccine control measures. Thanks to unrelenting vaccination campaigns, by 1977 only a few hundred cases existed in the world, in remote areas of Somalia, and health authorities were virtually certain that these would be the last cases of the once dreaded disease ever, anywhere.

An essential step in any method for the control of virus diseases is proper diagnosis. To be sure, the symptoms of some virus diseases are virtually unique, and when they appear, there is little question of the identity of the causative virus. For example, when the salivary glands of the jaw swell, the disease is almost certain to be mumps. But, often, diagnosis on the basis of symptoms alone is not possible. Even with mumps, the telltale jaw-swelling sometimes does not appear, and then the disease may be very difficult to diagnose. Under such circumstances, the physician turns to the clinical laboratory for help.

In general, laboratory diagnosis of viral diseases depends on one of two processes: isolation of the viruses themselves or detection of a rise in antibodies to the virus. To find viruses, samples are drawn of blood tissue, saliva, and so on, the choice depending on the nature of the symptoms. These samples are then placed in a situation in which the viruses can multiply and reveal their presence. They may, for instance, be injected into the brains of newborn mice, inserted into fertile hens' eggs, or mixed with the cells in tissue cultures. The resultant signs of disease or cell destruction show that a virus is at work; often their particular character pinpoints the virus. If not, the tests can be repeated, but now with antibodies to known viruses; the antibody that blocks the viral action is the antibody to that virus.

Blood levels of antibodies to viruses are determined by *serologic tests* using standard samples of clearly identified viruses. When infection by a certain virus is suspected, a test for antibodies to that virus is run as soon as possible, with a second test a week or so later. A fourfold rise in the level of antibodies between the two is taken to be indicative of infection by the virus in question.

It is difficult to summarize in a few pages everything that is known about virus diseases and the methods for detecting and controlling them. What has been said here gives only a bird's-eye view of that extremely varied terrain—as the entries that follow will show.

ACUTE IDIOPATHIC POLYNEURITIS. See GUILLAIN-BARRÉ SYNDROME.

ADENOVIRUS INFECTION. See RESPIRATORY INFECTION.

ALASTRIM. See SMALLPOX.

ALS. See AMYOTROPHIC LATERAL SCLEROSIS.

AMYOTROPHIC LATERAL SCLEROSIS (ALS). A not uncommon, chronic disease of the nervous system, amyotrophic lateral sclerosis causes weakness of various muscles, which gradually worsens and culminates in paralysis. The disease is almost invariably fatal, usually within two to six years. It is sometimes referred to as "Lou Gehrig's disease," after the popular American baseball player who died of it in 1941. (In the past it was often called "Charcot's disease" or "Charcot's syndrome," for the French neurologist who first described it.) Although the evidence is scanty, the disease may belong in the newly recognized category of SLOW VIRUS DISEASE.

Three out of four victims of amyotrophic lateral sclerosis are men, generally in the age group 50 to 60. According to some estimates as many as 10,000 new cases of the disease occur in the world each year.

This disease and several variants of it—progressive muscular atrophy, primary lateral sclerosis, and progressive bulbar palsy—affect different parts of the brain and spinal cord, producing varied patterns of symptoms. But the primary attack in each case is on the motor neurons—the nerve cells that regulate movement—and these conditions together are called "motor-neuron" or "motor-system" disease.

The symptoms begin with muscular weakness, tingling, or twitching, and pain or numbness. Knotting or cramping may also be noticed, along with muscle spasms. In time paralysis takes over.

Sometimes the first muscles hit are those of the tongue and throat, with the result that speaking and chewing are affected. More often the disease attacks the arms or legs first. Ultimately the disturbance extends to the trunk muscles. Death results from paralysis of the breathing apparatus or from a pneumonia caused indirectly by impairment of that function.

Throughout, the mind remains clear, and the senses acute. There is no cure, but symptomatic treatment makes the patient more comfortable and may delay the onset of paralysis.

It is chiefly by analogy with other degenerative nervous system

7

diseases (such as SUBACUTE SCLEROSING PANENCEPHALITIS) that a virus cause is suspected. No virus has been found in patients to date.

ANKYLOSING SPONDYLITIS. See CONNECTIVE TISSUE DISEASE.

ARBOVIRUS DISEASE. Of the great many known arboviruses—that is, viruses carried by insects or other arthropods*—only a few attack man. These produce a variety of illnesses, ranging from mild, sporadic, feverish disorders to terrifying, often fatal, tropical plagues.

There are some 200-odd known arbovirus infections, but two-thirds of these affect only animals, wild or domestic. Of those that trouble man, just some two dozen do so on any regular basis, and of these, only three are passed directly from man to man by their arthropod *vector*. These are YELLOW FEVER, DENGUE, and SANDFLY FEVER. The rest infect man merely as a dead-end offshoot from their usual cycle of animal to arthropod and back to animal again.

Four categories of arthropods act as vectors for arboviruses: mosquitoes, midges, sandflies, and ticks. All these are insects except ticks, which belong to the related order Arachnida. Typically the virus is drawn up by the vector with the host's blood as it feeds. Once inside the body of the vector, the virus multiplies, travels to the salivary glands, and is deposited in the blood of the next animal the vector feeds upon. Some arboviruses pass from one generation of the vector to the next via the eggs, with the result that offspring become infected without ever feeding on an infected host, but this is not usually the case.

Because of their mode of transmission, arboviruses must induce a state of *viremia* in their animal hosts, or the virus particles will not be picked up by the vector when it withdraws blood for feeding. Most arbovirus infections in man do not produce a sufficiently heavy viremia, or one of sufficiently long duration, for the virus to be spread in this way. Those that do, of course, are the three named above.

Almost all known animals act as hosts for one arbovirus or another, including many species of birds, as well as bats, mice, rats, rabbits, squirrels, chipmunks, sheep, cattle, and horses. Many of these animals act as hosts for viruses that also occasionally infect man.

Within the body of the host animal, human or otherwise, the virus— which has been conveniently inserted directly into the bloodstream by the

---

*The original contraction for "arthropod-borne virus" was "arborvirus," but this term was replaced by the present form, when it was realized that the older version seemed to describe a virus that invaded trees.

vector—multiplies in certain blood cells, producing what is generally a brief, transient viremia. It may then concentrate its attack on particular organs or tissues, most commonly the central nervous system, the small capillaries of the skin, or such internal organs as the liver and kidneys. According to how the virus behaves in the body it produces any of four disease patterns: (1) a mild, feverish illness, possibly with headache and nausea, corresponding largely to a state of viremia; (2) a more serious disorder marked by weakness, jaundice, and other signs of liver malfunction; (3) an ENCEPHALITIS or MENINGITIS indicating a disturbance of the central nervous system; or (4) skin rashes and bleeding from the mucous membranes and internal organs, a complex known as HEMOR-RHAGIC FEVER.

One striking feature of most arbovirus diseases is that there are a large number of *inapparent infections,* and when symptoms do occur, even in the normally more severe diseases, they often take the form only of the mild, feverish illness described above. This feverish illness is essentially all that is observed in the cases of sandfly fever, COLORADO TICK FEVER, and RIFT VALLEY FEVER. At the other extreme is yellow fever, the most fearsome of the arbovirus diseases. Very often fatal, it is marked by jaundice and heavy liver damage, with extensive internal bleeding. The many viral encephalitises—including the CALIFORNIA, ST. LOUIS, EQUINE, and TICK-BORNE ENCEPHALITISES—carry symptoms ranging from headache, drowsiness, and irritability, to coma, convulsions, and death. The hemorrhagic fevers, including dengue, also range considerably in severity—from mild rashes to severe and some-times fatal internal bleeding. Occasionally the kidney is hard hit, and kidney failure results.

Technically, the arboviruses are classified in groups, each containing viruses thought to be related because they cause similar *antibodies* to form in their animal hosts. The so-called A group includes the equine encephalitis viruses; three dengue-like viruses—the Mayaro, chikun-gunya, and o'nyong-nyong viruses (see DENGUE); two viruses that produce only inapparent infections or mild fevers in man—the Sindbis and Semliki Forest viruses; and a dozen or so animal viruses. Group B includes the yellow fever and true dengue viruses; the St. Louis en-cephalitis viruses (including West Nile fever virus, see DENGUE); the tick-borne encephalitis viruses; the hemorrhagic fever viruses; a group of viruses producing only fevers in man—the Kunjin virus of Australia and four African viruses, Spondwemi, Uganda S, Wesselsbron, and Zika; and again some dozen animal viruses. Group C and the Bunyamwera group, named for a representative member, consist of another dozen viruses each, most of which apparently infect only animals, though an occasional case of human fever is traced to one of these viruses. Other, smaller groups include the California encephalitis viruses; the sandfly fever viruses; several groups of viruses from Africa and South America that are of negligible importance in human disease, namely the Bwamba, Guama, and Simbu groups; and an assortment of ungrouped viruses, including the Colorado tick fever and Rift Valley fever viruses.

Formerly listed as a small group of arboviruses were the Tacaribe viruses, which cause hemorrhagic fever, and the LASSA FEVER virus. These viruses, however, are not carried by vectors, and now have been provisionally placed in a new group, the arenaviruses, along with the LYMPHOCYTIC CHORIOMENINGITIS virus, to which they are related.

Considering that they are classified together only because they happen to be carried by arthropods, the arboviruses show surprising similarity. All, for example, are *RNA* viruses, and most consist of moderately sized *icosahedral* particles, 40 to 60 nanometers in diameter (about two millionths of an inch), surrounded by an *outer envelope*. All have the ability to clump, or agglutinate, red blood cells of day-old chicks and geese, and tests based on this property are used to detect arboviruses in blood and tissue samples. *Serologic tests* based on the same property serve to detect antibodies to these viruses in the blood. The arboviruses themselves can also be observed by injecting suspect material into the brains of suckling mice. In positive tests, signs of encephalitis appear within five days. Infected mouse brains also are a rich source of viruses for study, and viruses are grown in hens' eggs and in *tissue cultures*. Vaccines for only a few arboviruses have been prepared; Max Theiler's yellow fever vaccines, which date from the 1930s, are the best known.

ARTERIOSCLEROSIS. See HEART DISEASE.

ARTHRITIS (RHEUMATISM). Formerly known in the United States as "rheumatism" (and still commonly designated by that term in Great Britain),* arthritis is a chronic, generally lifelong disorder of the joints. Characterized by pain, swelling, stiffness, and sometimes immobility or gross deformation, this condition is mainly, though not exclusively, one of middle or old age. Typically it follows an uneven course, with

---

*Usually now in the United States "rheumatism" is taken to be aches and pains in the muscles, tendons, and bones, possibly including the joints, but not limited to them, as arthritis is.

improvement often noted over long periods, but with a gradual worsening nonetheless. With careful medical management the patient is often fully functional and relatively pain- and symptom-free for much of the time, though he cannot be completely cured. Although the cause of arthritis has not yet been definitely established, there is some evidence that a virus may be involved, perhaps indirectly. Almost certainly arthritis is not a typical virus disease, which can be "caught" like a cold.

The world's major crippling disorder, arthritis, in one form or another, eventually hits nearly everyone: studies show that 97 percent of all people over the age of 60 have enough arthritis for it to show in X rays, even though a great many of them do not actually feel discomfort. It is estimated that 50 million Americans currently have some measure of joint disease, 20 million enough to require medical care. And every year 600,000 new cases are added to the rolls. The Arthritis Foundation—which supplies these figures—estimates that in the United States alone the disease causes an overall economic drain of $13 billion, due to lost time, money spent on drugs, and so on. Finally, whereas the young are generally thought to be spared the ravages of this disease, about 250,000 Americans suffer from the so-called juvenile arthritis, which strikes at any time from infancy to the teens.

Because of its effects on the bones arthritis is one of the oldest identifiable diseases. The skeleton of a Neanderthal man, dating from about 40,000 B.C., shows signs of arthritis. And dinosaurs from some 100 million years ago also seem to have suffered from it.

There are a number of forms of arthritis, and these may come to be recognized as quite different diseases, with different causes. In fact, the disorders commonly lumped together as arthritis actually are members of a larger family of more or less closely related diseases often designated CONNECTIVE TISSUE DISEASE. The chief forms of arthritis are osteoarthritis, rheumatoid arthritis, and juvenile rheumatoid arthritis. In the past, still another form of arthritis, that caused by bacterial infection, was relatively common. Mostly involved here were the bacteria that cause gonorrhea, pneumonia, and tuberculosis, as well as the staphylococci and streptococci ("staph" and "strep"). Now that bacterial infections are so well controlled by antibiotics, however, arthritis of this kind has all but disappeared.

Osteoarthritis is the most common type of arthritis, but also the mildest. Some two-thirds of all victims have this variety of the disease, which consists chiefly of breakdown of the cartilage in one or several joints. Whereas there may be considerable pain, and the joint may become difficult to use—and finally may even be completely immobilized—there is little inflammation and the disease is not *systemic*. This is the sort of arthritis that may show up only on X-ray examination.

With many patients, osteoarthritis just seems to be the result of wear and tear on the joint. It may be simply one of the many manifestations of aging and may not be fully understood until we have a better idea of what that process consists of. Sometimes it is larger joints that are hit, and particularly those that receive the most use—baseball pitchers get it in the elbow of the throwing arm, football players in the knees. But often osteoarthritis appears in the small joints of the fingers and toes. When this happens—and it seems to in women more than men—it usually does so at a relatively early age, perhaps around 40. A peculiarity of arthritis of the fingers is the development of large bumpy nodules—called Heberden's nodes when they occur on the first joints and Bouchard's nodes when they come on the second.

Rheumatoid arthritis is another matter. It is severe—painful and, unless carefully managed, highly crippling. A systemic, or body wide, disorder, it is characterized by generalized illness and localized inflammation in one, or more frequently many, joints. Typically a disease of middle age—actually, it commonly strikes first at any time between 20 and 50—rheumatoid arthritis hits twice as many women as men. Although it accounts for only about one quarter of all arthritis cases, these are generally the most serious.

As a rule, rheumatoid arthritis begins with fatigue and a diffuse soreness, stiffness, and aching in the joints. There is a loss of appetite and over a period of time a gradual decrease in weight. The hands and feet may be cold and sweaty. Sometimes the eyes become inflamed, and the patient may develop pleurisy or anemia. Finally, symptoms localize in particular joints, which swell up and become both warm and tender to the touch. After a short time the initial attack may subside—with the affected joints returning effectively to normal—and in a few cases the disease may never resume. Most of the time, however, the attack returns, and in time the joint involvement becomes continuous. Although the progress of the disease is uneven, the patient's ability to move the joints is increasingly diminished, first by pain, then by a stiffness that may completely immobilize a joint or badly deform it. Fingers, for example, may be so twisted out of line as to make grasping difficult.

What happens within the joint is well documented. The process begins with inflammation of the membrane that encloses the joint. Then a layer of fresh tissue begins to form, working its way between the ends of the bones that meet in the joint, and eroding away the cartilage that coats the bone ends. With the bone unprotected by cartilage, outgrowths of it extend into the new tissue, ultimately bridging and fusing the joint.

Juvenile rheumatoid arthritis occurs in two forms, a rather mild one, which develops slowly and almost always disappears with no after-effects, and a sudden, severe form, called Still's disease, which can be crippling if not treated promptly. (Paradoxically, Still's disease also occurs in adults.) Besides the usual arthritis symptoms, victims of Still's disease usually have a transient skin rash, their lymph glands swell, and the spleen may become inflamed. A retardation of growth in children is sometimes observed. The most serious complication is inflammation of the iris, which without proper treatment can lead to blindness.

In fact, with each type of arthritis, prompt and accurate diagnosis is important if crippling effects are to be minimized. The patient himself can be alerted by what the Arthritis Foundation lists as the arthritis warning signs: "persistent pain and stiffness on arising; pain, tenderness or swelling in one or more joints; recurrence of these symptoms, especially when they involve more than one joint; recurrent or presistent pain and stiffness in the neck, lower back, knees, and other joints."

One of the first things the physician does is rule out the presence of bacteria in the affected joint. (If they are found, of course, they are eliminated with antibiotics.) Osteoarthritis and rheumatoid arthritis are distinguished by the signs of general illness—fatigue, fever, head-ache—and joint inflammation—swelling and heat—both of which appear in rheumatoid but not osteoarthritis. Other factors also point to rheumatoid arthritis: the development of hard, almond-shaped knobs, "nodules," under the skin near the elbow; the fact that the same joints on both sides of the body are usually involved and to the same extent; and the tendency toward early morning stiffness, which persists for a few hours after waking. With either type of arthritis, X-ray examination confirms damage to the joint, and blood tests, urine tests, and tests of the fluid contained in the joints all aid in diagnosis. One blood component, the so-called rheumatoid factor, is found exclusively in patient's suffering from rheumatoid arthritis. Still's disease patients are usually diagnosed on the basis of age and the sudden onset and special pattern of symptoms, as well as an absence of rheumatoid factor in the blood.

Treatment for arthritis depends, of course, on the nature and severity of the symptoms, as well as on the age and condition of the patient. First of all, drugs do help. Aspirin is the long established—and often surprisingly effective—remedy; it not only eases pain but, in the case of rheumatoid arthritis, reduces inflammation. Because high dosages of aspirin are required—dosages to which some people respond badly—it is essential that the amount taken be established by the physician. (In any case, arthritis is too serious a problem to be treated by the patient alone.)

Several new anti-inflammatory agents are available—namely, in-domethacin, ibuprofen, and phenylbutazone—and with some patients their use may be called for. But these are potent drugs, with side effects that may be significant, and they are generally not employed unless there are good reasons why aspirin cannot be used.

Anti-inflammatory steroids, chiefly cortisone and several closely re-lated substances, also have an important role to play in arthritis treatment—but they too can have serious side effects and must be used carefully. Most commonly now they are given by single-dose injections into inflamed joints. Long-term oral medication with steroids, though sometimes still resorted to, is avoided if possible.

Recent research on a new class of hormonelike materials, the prosta-glandins, suggests that they are somehow involved in inflammation, and drugs related to or affecting the prostaglandins may someday help fight arthritis. Finally, other agents now used occasionally are gold salts and certain antimalarial drugs. These substances are not anti-inflammatory agents, but for reasons not yet understood, they do have a favorable effect on arthritis patients. They also can cause undesirable effects, however, and the patient taking them must be watched by his physician.

Any arthritis therapy program is likely to include mild exercise to prevent affected joints from stiffening up. The application of heat, either by wet packs or with heat lamps, may reduce pain and render joints more easily mobile. Hydrotherapy may provide a combination of mild exercise and heat therapy. At crucial times splinting of joints may prevent malformation, and for extreme cases surgical correction of joint abnor-malities may be needed. Replacement of hopelessly damaged joints with artificial ones is sometimes possible as a last resort.

The big question, still largely unanswered, is what causes arthritis. Although osteoarthritis seems to be only an aspect of the aging process and to involve a breakdown of the joint tissue by wear, this may not be the full or final story. At the moment, however, interest centers on rheumatoid arthritis in both the adult and juvenile forms, because these are closer to what we usually mean by disease and may have preventable causes.

A crucial aspect of rheumatoid arthritis is the inflammatory response that occurs in the joints—the kind of response that the body makes to foreign substances, such as material it is allergic to or bacterial invaders. (Though bacterial arthritis is known, there are no bacteria in the joints of patients with rheumatoid arthritis.) Some few authorities feel that arthritis is a kind of allergic reaction to certain foods, and claim to have success in treating arthritis by eliminating such foods from the diet—in practice they begin with a fasting period and continue adding foods to the diet one at a time until symptoms reappear, presumably indicating what foods are responsible. Most informed opinion is against this view, however, and attributes the presumed success obtained with the diets to a temporary alleviation of arthritis symptoms frequently found to occur following fasts.

The prevailing view is that arthritis, like certain other diseases, is an attack of the body on itself—an inflammatory response directed against the body's own tissues, in this case those of the joints. Diseases believed to be of this type are often called autoimmune, meaning that they represent an attack of the immunity system against the body it supposedly protects.

Nonetheless, there is growing evidence that the inflammatory response of rheumatoid arthritis is provoked by outside invaders. In several experiments, material from inflamed arthritic joints has been injected into mice, which then themselves developed arthritis, suggesting (though not proving) the transfer of an infectious agent. And workers in several laboratories have claimed to have identified such agents as bacterialike materials, though these results are not considered to be conclusive. The evidence that viruses may be involved in rheumatoid arthritis is still only secondhand.

For instance, it seems notable that some GERMAN MEASLES patients, and some who have received German measles vaccine, suffer transient arthritis. Furthermore, patients with other virus diseases, chiefly serum HEPATITIS, MUMPS, and MONONUCLEOSIS, also occasionally experience passing symptoms of arthritis. Also, with acute juvenile arthritis, Still's disease, one study of a number of patients showed (by *serologic tests*) that in each case an infection by any of several different viruses had preceded the arthritis attack. The viruses involved were mainly coxsackie viruses (see COXSACKIE OR ECHO VIRUS INFECTION); but mumps, CHICKEN POX, and German measles viruses were also found.

Beginning in 1975, a research team at Yale University came to recognize an epidemic form of arthritis, which occurs annually in late summer or early fall in eastern Connecticut. Called Lyme arthritis after a town in the area, this disease shows signs that it is carried by an insect: cases occur only in insect season and in rather close proximity to one another, and some victims remember having been bitten by a tick shortly before the attack. The disease hits many children, but adults too are victims. Swelling and inflammation of the joints and a generalized illness with fever are the main symptoms. An expanding circular reddish rash in the area of the presumed bite is another sign of the disease. Although no causative agent has yet been identified, the agent is thought to be a tick-borne virus.

What these various circumstances relating viruses and arthritis show is that at times a number of viruses can produce the symptoms of arthritis in patients. Whether or not these or some as yet unknown virus actually cause the many cases of juvenile and adult rheumatoid arthritis is another matter. Here there is simply not enough evidence. Some authorities would classify arthritis as a type of SLOW VIRUS DISEASE, a lingering ailment in which the virus remains in the body for long periods, perhaps in a masked form. If this is so, the autoimmune aspect of the disease may also be explained. If the virus sets up some kind of close association with certain cells—here, obviously those of the affected joints—it may alter them enough so that the body fails to recognize them and attacks them as invaders.

Although the hypothesis that arthritis is a slow virus disease is just that—a hypothesis—it gives arthritis researchers a target to aim at, and proving or disproving the hypothesis may help solve the mystery that is arthritis. One encouraging note is that if rheumatoid arthritis is even indirectly caused by a virus, or viruses, it may be possible to develop a vaccine that will prevent it.

ASCENDING PARALYSIS. See GUILLAIN-BARRÉ SYNDROME.

ASTHMA. Although asthma is not thought to be an infectious disease but rather an allergic or functional impairment of the respiratory tract, asthmatic attacks can be triggered by infections, including viral infections. In asthma there is a failure of the blood to be properly oxygenated, either through improper circulation of the blood in the lungs or through blockage of the airways that lead into the lungs, the bronchi. The typical signs of an asthmatic attack are wheezing, coughing, gasping for breath, and a rapidly beating heart. Fortunately drugs are available to reduce the severity of asthma attacks, and desensitization procedures decrease the likelihood of their being started by exposure to materials the patient is allergic to.

Whereas it is well documented that in many persons asthma attacks are initiated by allergies, in some individuals, especially those who develop asthma in middle age or later, there is no sign of allergic reaction. Even when allergy is present, it is likely that respiratory infections play a role, either in initiating attacks or complicating them. And in nonallergic asthma, it is suspected by some authorities that an infection is responsible for the underlying conditions. For a time it was assumed that only bacterial infection could stimulate or aggravate asthma attacks, but now it has been found that viral RESPIRATORY INFECTION too can do so. For asthmatics, then, it is advisable to avoid contact, whenever possible, with those suffering from respiratory virus infections.

AUSTRALIAN X DISEASE. See ST. LOUIS ENCEPHALITIS.

BELL'S PALSY. See HERPES.

BIRTH DEFECTS. See CYTOMEGALOVIRUS INFECTION, GERMAN MEASLES, HERPES.

BORNHOLM DISEASE. See PLEURODYNIA.

BOSTON EXANTHEM. See COXSACKIE OR ECHO VIRUS INFECTION.

BREAKBONE FEVER. See DENGUE.

BRONCHITIS. See RESPIRATORY INFECTION.

CALIFORNIA ENCEPHALITIS. California encephalitis (see ENCEPHALITIS) consists of a group of mild, mosquito-borne diseases, quite common in the United States, and also found in other parts of the Western Hemisphere and even Europe. Most cases are *inapparent,* but some illness does occur, especially in children. This may include anything from a slight fever with headache and stiff neck to full-blown encephalitis, marked by convulsions and coma. One death is recorded.

The best known member of the group, and perhaps the most persistent, is La Crosse encephalitis, which is found chiefly in a large area around La Crosse, Wisconsin. Annual epidemics occur there; in 1975, for example, there were 50 confirmed or suspected cases. The La Crosse virus was first isolated from the brain of a child who died of the disease in 1960—the only known fatality.

The first virus in the family was discovered in 1943 in mosquitoes in Kern County, California; at the time there were local cases of encephalitis, but the connection between the virus and the disease was not definitely made. Since then antibodies to this virus have been detected many times in the blood of California residents, but there is still little evidence to link the virus with actual disease. Related viruses have subsequently been found in Texas, Colorado, Montana, North Dakota, and Florida, as well as Canada, Trinidad, Brazil, Czechoslovakia, Yugoslavia, and Mozambique.* In most cases the viruses have been identified but their connection with human disease is not well established.

When severe cases of the disease do occur, as has been documented in Wisconsin, symptoms begin suddenly with headache and fever, followed in a day or two by convulsions, coma, and partial paralysis. Fever and mental confusion may persist for a week to 10 days, and recovery, though complete, is likely to be slow. In milder cases, symptoms may not extend beyond headache, fever, vomiting, and stiff neck, and these signs generally disappear within a day or two. That the vast majority of infections are inapparent is indicated by the large numbers of persons, especially adults, who carry *antibodies* to one of the viruses in this family but have suffered no identifiable illness.

Although the evidence is not complete, it seems to be the case that all these viruses are transported by mosquitoes and infect chiefly small wild animals. (Unlike the viruses of other encephalitises, these apparently do not make use of birds as hosts.) In Wisconsin the guilty mosquito has been identified as Aedes triseriatus, chiefly a forest dweller, which lays its eggs in water-filled holes in the base of trees (or in abandoned tires or tin cans). The animals involved are gray squirrels and chipmunks. In California the mosquitoes are Culex tarsalis and Aedes melanimon, and the suspect animals are rabbits, field mice, and ground squirrels.

Mild cases of the disease require little treatment beyond bed rest; severe cases call for hospitalization, and physicians are especially alert to the development of pressure on the brain should inflammation become severe. There are no vaccines, and control is best accomplished by mosquito eradication. Because of strictures against the use of insecticides, the identification and cleaning up of mosquito breeding sites is the most feasible approach.

Diagnosis is generally accomplished by detection of sharp rises of

---

*It is not clear whether the various viruses involved here represent separate strains of a single virus or closely related but discrete species. At any rate, the members of the family so far identified, besides the La Crosse and the original California strain, are as follows: trivittatus virus, found in North Dakota and Florida; San Angelo, from Texas; snowshoe hare, Montana and Ontario; Jamestown Canyon, Colorado; Jerry Slough, California; Keystone, Florida; Melao, Trinidad and Brazil; Tahyna, Czechoslavakia and Yugoslavia; and Lumbo, Mozambique.

antibodies to the viruses during the course of infection. For this purpose *serologic tests* are run as soon as possible after the appearance of symptoms and again in one to three weeks. A fourfold rise in antibodies is taken to be a sign of active infection. In fatal cases, sample of brain tissue can be injected into suckling mice, in which the virus produces a quickly fatal encephalitis.

The viruses in the group are among the general class of arboviruses (see ARBOVIRUS DISEASE). The virus particles themselves are *icosahedral*, have a diameter of about 50 nanometers (two millionths of an inch), and are surrounded by an *outer envelope*.

CANCER. One of the most feared of all diseases, cancer is a disorder in which various body cells become abnormal, or malignant, often forming tumors that not only invade the surrounding tissues but also travel to new sites in the body, "metastasize." The most insidious feature of the disease is that, left to itself, it is almost inevitably fatal. Surgery, chemotherapy, and radiation are all used to treat cancer, with varying degrees of success, depending on (1) the type of cancer, (2) the number, size, and location of the tumors, and (3) the age, health, and genetic makeup of the patient. Many things are known to initiate cancer: injury, radiation, certain chemicals called carcinogens, and—definitely in animals, probably in man—viruses. Exactly how these various agents function in causing cancer in not known, though scientists have many ideas; nor is it known whether or not they all operate to cause cancer through a single mechanism.

Cancer may be as old as man: there are signs of cancer in Egyptian mummies. The ancient Greeks knew the disease and called it "karkinos," meaning crab. ("Cancer" is the Latin version of the same word, used also for the zodiacal sign.) Presumably this name reflects either the physical appearance of the tumor or its tenacious grip on the body.

Because cancer affects so many different tissues and organs of the body, and because it renders them malignant to such varying degrees, a single and typical case of cancer does not exist; cancer is often said to be not one disease but a hundred. Whereas ordinary skin cancer is slow growing and not prone to extensive metastasis, certain cancers of the internal organs develop so quickly that death may ensue in a matter of months. The experience of each cancer patient is virtually unique.

Probably as a reflection of differing life-styles and genetic endowments, the peoples of the world have quite different incidences of the various kinds of cancer. In Japan and Iceland, for example, there is twice as much stomach cancer as in the rest of the world. Overall, women experience slightly more cancer than men, due probably to the sensitivity to cancer of the breasts and uterus. Although cancer tends to hit at middle age or later, it can strike at any time. Also, the incidence of any one type of cancer often changes dramatically with time. Lung cancer in men, for instance, has increased twenty fold in the last 40 years (reflecting, many authorities believe, increases in cigarette smoking).

The ease of detection of cancers depends on their location: those at or near the surface of the body may be readily visible, whereas those associated with the internal organs may make their presence known only as they cause changes in body functions. The American Cancer Society lists seven warning signs of cancer: changes in bowel or bladder habits, a sore that does not heal, unusual bleeding or discharge, thickening or a lump in the breast or elsewhere, indigestion or difficulty in swallowing, obvious change in a wart or mole, and a nagging cough or hoarseness. At the persistence of any of these signs for more than two weeks, the patient is advised to see a physician. Experience has shown that any cancer is most successfully treated in the early stages of its development.

In order to complete his diagnosis, the physician will rely on physical examination, X-ray studies, and the use of special instruments (such as the proctoscope) for peering into the recesses of the body. To identify certain types of cancer such as myeloma, he will employ blood tests. A newer, still experimental method of cancer diagnosis is thermography, the use of a heat-detecting instrument, which finds cancers as hot spots among the normal body tissues. The final confirmatory test for cancer is always the examination of cells under the microscope to determine whether or not they are cancerous. Often such cells are taken by biopsy or during exploratory surgery, but in some cases, such as in the "Pap" test for cervical cancer, free cells may be obtained in the body secretions.

Surgery, cutting away of the tumor, is the oldest and most frequently employed method of cancer treatment; it is most successful when the tumor is small and has not metastasized. Irradiation with X rays or the emissions of radioactive elements (radium, cobalt-60) can be used to supplement or replace surgery. With leukemia, for example, a cancer of the white blood cells, there is no solid tumor to be removed surgically. Fortunately, leukemia and a related disorder, Hodgkin's disease, respond well to radiation therapy, as well as to the third form of cancer treatment, chemotherapy. Some tumors, such as those of the prostate, can be controlled with administered hormones—a kind of chemotherapy—but most chemotherapeutic agents are highly toxic substances. (Some of them are related to the mustard gas of World War I.) Since these agents operate generally by being more toxic to cancer cells than they are to normal ones, they must be employed with much caution. In use, they are sometimes accompanied by painful and debilitating side effects.

Recently, scientists have begun to experiment with a new method of cancer treatment: immunotherapy, or stimulation of the immunity system so that it can itself better fight off the cancer. One way this is done is with a type of tuberculosis vaccine, bacillus Calmette-Guérin (BCG), which is known to stimulate the immune system. Certain drugs, such as the substance levamisole, are also thought to act in this way, and several of them—including levamisole—have been tested successfully against cancers.

With various combinations of these methods, physicians have mixed success in treating cancers. Some, like leukemia, Hodgkin's disease, and choriocarcinoma (a rare tumor in women that arises from the placenta), respond well to treatment—many victims of these cancers have, after treatment, essentially normal lifespans. Many other tumors, however, are unresponsive to treatment, and the outlook for those who develop them is bleak.

Because of the somewhat limited success of conventional cancer therapy—and the often severe side effects of certain forms of it—quack cancer cures have long been a medical problem. Often such supposed remedies are themselves harmless, but they raise false hopes, drain large sums of money from frightened families, and above all prevent cancer patients from seeking legitimate therapy. In recent years most controversy has centered on the substance laetrile, an extract of apricot pits, which is said to release cyanide in the body. This substance has been repeatedly tested against cancer and found ineffective—though proponents of the drug contest the adequacy of the tests. With the support of the National Cancer Institute and the American Cancer Society, the Food and Drug Administration has condemned the drug and banned its sale in the United States, but a number of states have passed laws legalizing the drug. The matter is now being fought out in the courts.

It has been known for a long time that repeated, small irritations, such as those from an ill-fitting denture, can lead to cancer at the affected site, but it is generally considered unlikely that a single blow or injury can do so. That certain chemicals can cause cancer also has been understood for a long time—in 1775 an English surgeon, Percivall Pott, suggested that chimney sweeps developed skin cancer because of their constant exposure to soot. In the 20th century a number of specific chemicals have been identified as carcinogens, and the list of such substances grows steadily longer. Radiation too can cause cancer, as became clear soon after the discovery of X rays and the first isolation of radium. Madame Curie, discoverer of radium, herself died of leukemia from exposure to radiation, and in the 1920s many workers who painted radium numerals on watches developed bone cancer.

It is thought by most authorities that these physical and chemical agents account for most cases of human cancer—at least 80 percent, possibly much more. Several questions remain, however: Do viruses cause any of the remaining cases? And is there some common bond that links these various cancer-causing processes?

The first evidence connecting viruses to cancers in animals was reported in 1911, when Peyton Rous of the Rockefeller Institute described his discovery of what is now known as the Rous chicken sarcoma virus. (It is indicative of the reaction of the scientific community to Rous's discovery that he received the Nobel Prize in Medicine for it—in 1966!) Since 1911, ample evidence has accumulated that many different viruses can cause cancer in animals, and there is good—though not conclusive—evidence that viruses are responsible for at least four different kinds of human cancer: Burkitt's lymphoma, cancer of the uterine cervix, certain kinds of leukemia, and mammary cancer.

The human cancer that seems most certainly to be virus-caused is Burkitt's lymphoma, a cancer of the lymph glands of the jaw, first observed in African children in the 1950s by a British surgeon, Denis Burkitt. The disease occurs mainly in a geographically limited region of Africa, where Burkitt happened to be stationed, although isolated cases are found from time to time in other parts of the world. By studying the distribution of African cases, Burkitt concluded that an infectious agent must be involved, possibly a virus carried by mosquitoes—maps showing the distribution of cases coincided closely with those showing the incidence of malaria.

In 1964 two virologists working in London, M. A. Epstein and Yvonne Barr, found a virus in a *tissue culture* prepared from cells from the tumor of a Burkitt's lymphoma patient. Subsequently, other investigators have found the virus in cells from other Burkitt's lymphoma patients. Moreover, they have detected the presence of *DNA* from the virus (virus genes) in tumor cells from a great many such patients, and they have found *antibodies* to the virus in the patients' blood. Furthermore, it is found that the virus is able to transform normal white blood cells in cultures until they come to resemble lymphoma cells. And, finally, investigators have injected monkeys with such transformed cells and with the Epstein-Barr virus itself, and in both cases have observed the formation of malignant lymphomas.

Similar studies, though not as complete, link the Epstein-Barr virus with Hodgkin's disease and with nasopharyngeal carcinoma, a cancer of the nose and throat, which is extremely rare except among the Chinese. In none of these cases does the evidence prove that the Epstein-Barr virus is responsible for the cancer, but the implication, especially with respect to Burkitt's lymphoma, is very strong.

On the other hand, in the period since its discovery, the Epstein-Barr virus, which is related to the HERPES or cold-sore virus, has been found to be rather common. Most adults carry antibodies to it, suggesting that they have been exposed at one time or another, though they may never have had an ailment attributable to the virus. The disease the virus seems to be responsible for is MONONUCLEOSIS—patients with the disease show a rise of antibodies to the virus. But mononucleosis patients are not especially susceptible to Burkitt's lymphoma, Hodgkin's disease, or nasopharyngeal carcinoma. Thus, it seems clear that nearly everyone is exposed to the Epstein-Barr virus, with some developing mononucleosis as a result, but with only a minute percentage of those exposed developing cancer. Why this should be is a great mystery. In Africa, it is suggested, a second infectious agent may be involved in the cases of Burkitt's lymphoma, possibly malaria, which seems to have an effect on the body's cellular immunity system and could in that way be setting the stage for the action of the virus.

Another herpes virus that is strongly implicated in human cancer is the so-called herpes-2 virus. This virus very much resembles its cousin, the ordinary herpes virus, but it infects the genital area rather than the mouth. Much evidence now links this virus with cervical cancer—a rather common malignancy, which affects 90,000 American women a year.

The first indication that cervical cancer might be caused by a transmissible agent came from findings that the disorder was more common in women who had multiple sex partners. Subsequently, a statistical correlation was found between cervical cancer and venereal infection by the herpes-2 virus. (Such a correlation indicated only a relationship—that is, that the two variables tend to occur together—but not necessarily a causal one.) According to one such study, women with antibodies to the herpes-2 virus are eight times as likely to develop cervical cancer as women without. Obviously, not every woman with genital herpes develops cervical cancer, but the odds are quite high—as many as six out of a hundred may do so, according to some estimates.

There is other evidence. Abnormal, "precancerous" cervical cells have been observed in mice experimentally infected with herpes-2 virus, and mouse cells grown in tissue culture have been transformed by the virus into cells capable of causing tumors when injected into live mice.

Also, newborn hamsters have developed malignant tumors after being injected with the virus. In addition, herpes viruses have been obtained from a line of cells cultured from a human cervical carcinoma. Finally, several studies have purported to show the presence of herpes virus DNA in cervical cancer cells (and cells of other kinds of tumors possibly caused by herpes viruses), but this work has been difficult to repeat.

Normally, herpes viruses destroy cells in tissue culture without transforming them into cancer cells, and transformation is achieved only by first inactivating the viruses. One way of doing this is by treating them with certain dyes and then exposing them to light. This same process had been proposed as a way of inactivating herpes viruses in the body and thereby stopping infections, but the fact that the process can cause cancerous cell transformation in the laboratory strongly calls its use in human beings into question.

In addition to the evidence connecting herpes-2 virus with cervical cancer, there is some indication that it may cause penile cancer, which is rather rare, and possibly even prostatic cancer, which is far more common. Similarly, the herpes-1 virus—the ordinary cold sore virus—is suspected of having cancer-causing potential. Cancer of the lip, the most likely prospect, is most uncommon, but the virus could conceivably cause cancers of the mouth, throat, and nose—possibly even those at more remote sites.

Whereas virologists have only strong suspicions that the herpes-2 virus and the Epstein-Barr virus cause cancers in human beings, they have conclusive evidence that other herpes viruses cause several different kinds of cancer in animals. One such virus, dubbed the Lucké virus after the researcher who discovered it, causes kidney cancers in frogs; others are responsible for lymphomas in rabbits, cattle, and guinea pigs. Furthermore, two much studied monkey herpes viruses lead to tumors when injected into a monkey of a species other than those they normally infect.

But the cancer-causing herpes virus of most interest is that of Marek's disease, a disorder of chickens, which causes great loss of life, chiefly from lymphomas. The most significant feature of this disease is that virologists have developed a vaccine against it, the only known cancer vaccine. Although the vaccine—which is based on an *attenuated virus* grown in turkeys—does not altogether halt the multiplication of the virus in chickens, it does prevent the formation of tumors.

Needless to say, the existence of such a vaccine is important because it suggests the feasibility of comparable vaccines that might halt the development of herpes virus-induced tumors in people. In fact, work on such vaccines is already underway. One has been successfully tested in monkeys, another reportedly in human beings.

But herpes viruses are not the only viruses known to cause cancers in animals and suspected of doing so in people. The other major group of cancer viruses is the oncornaviruses—the name indicates a tumor-producing capacity ("oncos" is a Greek word for tumor) and the fact that the viruses contain RNA. There are two kinds of oncornaviruses, known as B-type and C-type, which are differentiated by their appearance in the electron microscope. (The C-type are symmetrical, the B-type assymmetrical.)

Actually, the C-type viruses were discovered first. In fact, the first tumor virus of all, the Rous chicken sarcoma virus, is in this category. The C-type oncornaviruses cause sarcomas—a particular class of solid tumor—and also leukemia in a wide variety of mammals and birds. A great deal of research has been done on the animal C-type viruses, and the picture is a somewhat confusing one. To begin with, the C-type leukemia viruses multiply in cultured cells without transforming them into cancer cells, whereas the sarcoma viruses (which are said to be defective) transform the cells without producing new viruses. And when both viruses infect cells together, virus particles of both kinds are produced and the cells are transformed. To complicate the picture even further, many inbred animals carry so-called endogenous viruses of the C-type; such viruses appear to have become an almost normal part of the animal's cells and are passed on from generation to generation. Although endogenous viruses normally do not cause cancer in their hosts, they are sometimes activated in such a way that they do so.

There is increasingly good evidence that C-type oncornaviruses are involved in human leukemia, possibly also in human sarcoma. First of all, the particles can be observed in electron micrographs of human leukemia and sarcoma cells. But the same, or very similar, particles can be observed—though less frequently—in comparable cells from normal patients.

More convincing evidence concerns an enzyme carried by the particles of all oncornaviruses. This enzyme has been called a "reverse transcriptase" because it reverses the normal procedure and transcribes genetic information from RNA to DNA. A reverse transcriptase that much resembles the one in animal C-type viruses has been found in human leukemia cells. Also, there is evidence of certain nucleic acids related to those in animal C-type viruses in human leukemia cells but not normal cells.

And, finally, after many earlier premature announcements that human

C-type viruses had been found, in 1975 cancer researchers cautiously suggested that several such particles actually had been isolated from the cells of leukemia patients. Earlier supposed isolations had proved to be animal viruses derived from cells the viruses had been transferred to. Such a possibility seemed to have been ruled out in the new cases, but having been mistaken before, scientists were proceeding slowly.

That any such C-type viruses in leukemic cells are not endogenous is suggested by research with identical twins, one with leukemia, and one not. The finding is that cells from the twin with leukemia contain viral nucleic acid, whereas those from the normal twin do not.

Human B-type oncornaviruses are also thought to be responsible for some cases of cancer, but here the evidence is less firm. It has been amply demonstrated that B-type viruses cause mammary cancer in mice and monkeys, but genetic factors are also involved. Thus, the same virus causes a great many tumors in mice of some inbred strains, none at all in those of others. Also, the viruses differ in the way they are transmitted. Sometimes the virus is passed on to the offspring in the mother's milk; at times it is transmitted in the seminal fluid of the male parent. With some viruses, the viral nucleic acid actually becomes incorporated into the nucleic acid of the ova or sperm cells and is transmitted from generation to generation like any other genetic material. In any case, the virus is present in virtually all animals of the strain, and whether or not cancer occurs depends on hormonal, dietary, and other factors.

In many human patients with breast cancer, B-type particles can be observed in tumor tissue, but they can also be found on occasion in normal breast tissue. Likewise, a reverse transcriptase enzyme similar to that from B-type animal viruses can be found in human milk samples— but not exclusively from women with any history of breast cancer (or any record of it in their immediate families). Unlike the case with mice of some strains, there is no evidence that women who have themselves been breast fed as infants are any more likely than other women to develop breast cancer.

The most positive finding relating B-type viruses to human breast cancer is the detection in cancer tissue of RNA and proteins very similar to those found in mouse B-type cancer viruses (but differing from those found in C-type viruses). Such RNA and proteins are not detected in normal tissue.

What many virologists now assume is that the B viruses are quite widespread, with many women harboring them, and that they are a necessary but not a sufficient condition for breast cancer development— that is, that they must be present if the cancer is to start, and indeed that they are themselves directly involved in the process, but that something else must also be present. The other factor that may be involved is hormone changes, which in mice seem to play a role in the cancer-initiation process. Although it looks very much as though such human viruses are not transmitted in the mother's milk, no one is quite sure exactly how they do get from person to person; perhaps they are endogenous viruses.

So there are suspicious circumstances linking at least four viruses with human cancer: the Epstein-Barr virus, the herpes-2 virus, and the B and C oncornaviruses. These putative connections suggest certain possibilities with respect to control of the particular cancers involved.

The herpes-2 virus is a somewhat special case. Here the presence of the virus is almost always signaled by a visible infection of the external genitalia. Although the infection is sometimes quiescent for long periods—as is herpes of the lips—when the outbreaks come they can generally be felt, as an itching or burning sensation, and seen, as tiny blisterlike sores.

It is quite clear that genital herpes is on the rise—some authorities speak of an epidemic—and the disease is especially troublesome because, once contracted, it seldom goes away. Yet there is hope. Some experimental drugs are highly effective in tests (see HERPES), though none is yet available for general use. And the success of the vaccine against Marek's disease raises expectations that a vaccine of some type might be developed for use against the herpes-2 virus.

Nonetheless, at present, women with genital herpes are clearly at some increased risk of developing cervical cancer. This does not in itself call for panic—only a small percentage of women with herpes-2 infections will actually get cancer. But the risk is there and such women are well advised to seek periodic gynecological examinations. Certainly, also, the physician should be informed about the herpetic condition—if it is in a quiescent state, it will not be observed. Fortunately cervical cancer is one that can be detected early—often a precancerous phase is observable—and with early treatment, it can generally be cured.

For men with herpes-2 infections, and for all those having herpes-1 infections, there is little to be alarmed about—the connection with cancer is extremely tenuous. Again, however, it is wise to inform the physician about the condition; the more he knows, the better he is able to do his job.

The Epstein-Barr virus, too, leads to an observable disease, mononu-cleosis, but only in small number of people exposed to the virus, and these people seem to be at no special risk of developing cancer. In fact, the fraction of people exposed to the Epstein-Barr virus who develop cancer is so minute that little thought is given to identifying those exposed.

For those who do develop cancers due to this virus, the outlook is not unfavorable. Burkitt's lymphoma is mainly limited to Africa, and the African cases have been found to respond very well to the cancer drug methotrexate. Nasopharyngeal carcinoma is rare and not considered a major health problem. Hodgkin's disease, on the other hand, while not common, does have a fairly high incidence, but it too responds quite well to drug treatment.

Over the long run, there is no reason to think that a vaccine could not be developed against the Epstein-Barr virus. Presumably, then, both mononucleosis and the cancers associated with the virus would disappear.

With the B and C oncornaviruses, prospects are somewhat less clear. Until more is known about the relation of these viruses to human cancer, it might seem that very little could be done in the way of prevention or treatment that was directed at the virus. Since there is some suspicion that both types of virus are endogenous—almost, if not quite, permanent parts of the human cell—vaccines against them might not be possible. Even if this is the case, however, the virus presumably must be activated in some way if it is to initiate cancer, and a vaccine directed at certain viral products or altered cell components conceivably could be of value. (In fact, the activation step could in some way be susceptible to interference by chemical agents, and that would render these cancers subject to chemotherapy.)

Paradoxically, some authorities believe that the best way to demonstrate that oncornaviruses do cause cancer in man would be to prepare vaccines against them and show that the vaccines prevent the suspect cancers. Workers with mouse mammary cancer viruses (B-type) have shown that vaccines can be effective in reducing incidence of tumors even in mice with endogenous viruses. (Better results are obtained with virus-free mice.) It has been suggested that a mouse virus vaccine might protect women against the human virus, just as vaccination with the cowpox virus protects againt SMALLPOX.

Generally, then, the likelihood that at least some cancers are caused by viruses is, all things considered, a hopeful sign. Viruses, after all, are a known quantity; over the years medical researchers have developed a number of ways of dealing with them: vaccines, chiefly, but now, it is hoped, many new drugs. Really effective control of virus-caused cancer, however—of all cancer, for that matter—may not come until scientists better understand how normal cells are converted to cancerous ones by viruses—and other agents.

There are many theories of how cancers get started, most of them having something to do with the nucleic acid, the DNA of the cell, which contains the essential information for regulating the life of the cell, and for duplicating it when the need arises. It seems almost certain that when a normal cell becomes cancerous, its DNA is in some way altered. The new, cancerous cell is able to pass its own malignant character on to its offspring cells, and this would seem to be possible only through the agency of the DNA.

Irritation, radiation, and chemical carcinogens are all thought to render cells cancerous by altering their DNA. Both carcinogens and radiation are known to have the potential for changing DNA inasmuch as they cause mutations, which are known to arise from alterations in DNA. And repair of repeated injuries involves continued proliferation of new cells and consequently almost constant replication of DNA, with enhanced possibilities for alteration in all the new DNA being formed.

Presumably, viruses too can alter cellular DNA. Some bacterial viruses, or bacteriophages, operate by inserting their DNA into that of the bacteria they invade, permanently altering the bacterial cells in the process. Conceivably, then, DNA cancer viruses could insert their DNA into that of the cells of their hosts, in some way causing them to become cancerous. There is, in fact, good evidence that certain animal cancer viruses do indeed cause their own DNA to become part of the DNA of the cells they make cancerous—viral DNA can actually be detected in the DNA of the tumor cells.

Even RNA cancer viruses could act in this way, by virtue of the reverse transcriptase enzyme they carry. With this enzyme a DNA equivalent of the viral RNA is prepared, and the new DNA could then make its way into the cellular DNA. Again, there is good evidence that such a process actually occurs with animal cancer viruses. Indeed, something very much like this probably happens with the endogenous oncornaviruses described above.

What happens when a virus causes cancer, then, is very different from what happens when it causes an ordinary disease. In the latter case, the virus invades certain cells of the body and multiplies within them, often destroying them in the process; the symptoms of disease are the result of that cell destruction. But when a virus causes cancer, it invades a great many body cells and renders only a very few of them cancerous. These cancer cells then proceed to grow and multiply on their own, producing the disease cancer in the body.

This picture of how viruses cause cancer explains why such cancers are not contagious in the usual sense. The virus is presumably a relatively common one to which most of us are exposed, but from which only a few individuals, in whom the conditions happen to be right, acquire cancer. The cancer itself cannot spread to new individuals, though the virus can—but the vast majority of those it infects will not develop cancer. The cancer virus itself, however, is still subject to the same control measures that affect other viruses.

With all cancers, the assumption that the cancer comes about from changes in the DNA does not really explain what alterations those DNA changes bring about in the cell. Possibly a control mechanism that prevents the cell from multiplying freely is blocked; possibly the surface of the cell is altered in such a way that the cell no longer responds properly to its environment. (There is some evidence supporting each of these hypotheses.) But, in any case, changes of some kind in the activity of the cell must come about, and it is these changes that may ultimately provide the key to the control of cancer. Once researchers understand what these changes are, perhaps they can develop specific ways of blocking them— and the methods they select could prove to be the more effective cancer control methods of the future.

CARDIOVASCULAR DISEASE. See HEART DISEASE.

CENTRAL ASIAN HEMORRHAGIC FEVER. See HEMORRHAGIC FEVER.

CENTRAL EUROPEAN ENCEPHALITIS. See TICK-BORNE EN-CEPHALITIS.

CHICKEN POX (VARICELLA). Chicken pox is a common, mild disease of early childhood, characterized by low fever and a pimply rash. In adults who have had the disease as children, it sometimes recurs in the form of the painful and protracted disorder SHINGLES.

Cases of chicken pox much resemble mild attacks of SMALLPOX, and for many centuries the distinction between the two diseases was not recognized. Nevertheless, the Sicilian physician Ingrassia clearly described chicken pox in 1553, and the Englishman William Heberden finally differentiated it from smallpox in the late 18th century.

The *incubation period* of chicken pox is about 2 weeks—though it may run anywhere from 11 to 21 days. The rash, which may or may not be preceded by a short period of fever and general illness, quickly develops into small pimples, then blisterlike pustules. After 3 or 4 days scabs have formed. The eruption is heaviest on the trunk of the body, with the face, arms, and legs more lightly attacked. It comes in successive waves, with the result that all stages of development may be present simultaneously. After 2 or 3 weeks the scabs fall away, leaving no scars.

Although most cases are uneventful and uncomplicated, EN-CEPHALITIS and pneumonia do sometimes occur, and bacterial infection of the sores is occasionally found. In children, especially, the disease is minor; in adults, who constitute about 20 percent of the cases, the general illness is more severe, and complications—pneumonia, in particular—more common.

The disease is highly contagious. It is probably spread by droplets emitted from the nose and throat and, more importantly, by direct contact with viruses shed from these areas or the skin sores. The sores have been said to contain little free virus, but the disease has been transmitted experimentally by inoculation of fluid withdrawn from them. The dried scabs, unlike those of smallpox, are not infectious. Little is known certainly about the movements of the virus within the body; presumably it enters through the mouth or respiratory tract, multiplies there and in the blood and internal organs, and is transported to the skin, where the obvious cell damage occurs.

Almost everyone not previously infected seems to be susceptible to chicken pox. Worldwide in scope, the disease is *endemic* in most large cities, and although there is no great regularity, outbreaks tend to occur in the winter. Because chicken pox is so contagious, most people experience it early, between the ages of two and eight. The disease gives lifelong immunity (except, of course, when it reappears as shingles), and reported second cases probably indicate original misdiagnoses.

The usual treatment is simply to keep infected children at home, give them aspirin if they have fever, and alleviate the itching that accompanies the rash with calamine lotion or drugs that specifically prevent itching. It is wise to minimize scratching because the sores become infected rather easily; when this occurs, however, antibiotics usually clear up the secondary infection promptly. With adults, bed rest may be called for. Development of encephalitis, signaled by headache, drowsiness, changes in behavior, and possible convulsions or lapses into coma, is rare and may pass quickly, but demands careful medical supervision. Pneumonia, characterized by increasing difficulty in breathing and a deepening cough, is a serious complication, especially in adults, and usually requires hospitalization. A serious and sometimes fatal form of chicken pox may develop in patients undergoing steroid therapy. For such patients, the therapy is usually discontinued temporarily when chicken pox is suspected; and steroid drugs are rarely given to chicken pox patients. Several new experimental drugs have been found to be active against the chicken pox virus, and their possible use in shingles is under investigation (see Shingles for a discussion). In time, such drugs may be called upon in more serious cases of chicken pox; normally there is no need.

Chicken pox is such a mild disease in most people that trying to prevent it is not worth the effort. Children who contract the disease are not isolated or quarantined, nor are other children encouraged to avoid them. In fact, it makes little sense to prevent infection in childhood only to postpone it to adulthood when it can be more severe. For people considered to be in special danger—such as those regularly taking cortisone, anticancer drugs, or drugs that prevent rejection of transplants—*gamma globulin* is given as a preventive measure after exposure. No vaccine has been developed, not only because of the mildness of the disease, but also because it is not clear whether the vaccinees would be likely to develop shingles in later life.

It usually is easy to diagnose chicken pox on the basis of symptoms alone—doubly so when the patient is known to have been exposed. Yet, confusion with other childhood rashes, or skin infections such as impetigo, does occur—even insect bites may sometimes be mistaken for chicken pox. Generally no harm is done by such misdiagnoses. More of a problem, however, is the occasional confusion of chicken pox with mild cases of smallpox, especially in previously vaccinated individuals. The highly contagious and serious nature of smallpox makes exact diagnosis mandatory—something that can be accomplished only in the laboratory.

Chicken pox and smallpox can be distinguished when properly stained material from the skin sores is examined under the microscope. Certain "giant" cells are found in chicken pox but not in smallpox. Furthermore, in smallpox so-called "elementary bodies" (in fact, the virus particles) are abundant and show up clearly; with chicken pox they are scarce and difficult to perceive. The two kinds of virus particles can also be differentiated under the electron microscope.

Chicken pox viruses can almost always be positively identified by laboratory tests with known *antibodies*. And, finally, sharp rises of antibodies to the virus, a clean sign of infection, can be detected (by *serologic tests*) in blood samples drawn when the first signs of illness appear, and again on convalescence.

The virus that causes chicken pox is a large one—about 200 nanometers in diameter (eight millionths of an inch). It consists of a central polyhedron containing a *DNA*-protein core and surrounded by an *outer envelope* with projecting spikes. The virus very much resembles the

HERPES virus, to which it is related. (The chicken pox virus is sometimes given the formal name "herpes varicella virus.") Although the chicken pox virus does not grow in laboratory animals or hens' eggs, it can be produced in *tissue cultures* of various types for laboratory study.

CHIKUNGUNYA VIRUS INFECTION. See DENGUE.

COLLAGEN DISEASE. See CONNECTIVE TISSUE DISEASE.

COLORADO TICK FEVER (MOUNTAIN FEVER). A mild, feverish illness lasting less than a week, Colorado tick fever occurs only in the wooded areas of the western United States during spring and early summer. The virus that causes the disease is normally carried by ground squirrels and is conveyed to man by the bite of the tick Dermacentor andersoni.

After an *incubation period* of three to six days, the symptoms appear—namely, fever and chills, headaches (with pain localized behind the eyes), bodily aches and pains, and nausea. Often the illness moderates after several days and then resumes for a few more days. When blood tests are run, a low white-cell count is found. Sometimes a rash occurs over the trunk and limbs, and on occasion a stiff neck and other signs of MENINGITIS are observed. In children the symptoms may be more severe. Usually recovery is rapid, even among children, and the patient is almost always back to normal within two weeks.

There is no special treatment for the disease, and no vaccine has been developed. Control can be accomplished only by tick eradication. So far, cases of the disease have occurred in Colorado, Utah, Nevada, California, Oregon, Washington, Idaho, Montana, Wyoming, and South Dakota, where the tick D. andersoni occurs naturally.

Laboratory diagnosis is by way of virus isolation from the blood—injection into suckling mice causes encephalitis—or by *serologic tests* performed early and late during the course of the disease. A fourfold rise in the level of *antibodies* to the virus is indicative of the disease. The virus appears to be a typical arbovirus (see ARBOVIRUS DISEASE).

THE COMMON COLD. Truly the most common, though hardly the most serious, of all diseases, the cold is a mild and short-lived—but troublesome—RESPIRATORY INFECTION. It occurs, or has occurred, at every spot on the globe. Although it is more frequently found in the temperate zones, it appears alike in tropical jungles and arctic wastes. Colds occur mainly in the fall, winter, and spring, but people get summer

colds too. Most adults average perhaps two or three colds a year—
varying expert opinion places this figure at anywhere from one to five—
and children have more. By their prevalence alone colds cause substantial
loss of working time and are a serious economic drain. In the United
States the cost of colds, including time off from work and money spent on
drugs and other medical care, is estimated at $3 billion. More impor-
tantly, of course, colds are a source of real discomfort to hundreds of
millions of people every year.

The common cold can be defined medically as "an acute, afebrile,
self-limited disease, characterized by nasal catarrh and pharyngeal irritation." This means that the disease comes on abruptly, is not usually
accompanied by fever, ends of its own accord, and causes chiefly a runny
nose and sore throat. It is but one of a number of more or less similar
respiratory disorders, which are differentiated more by the nature of the
symptoms than by the causative agent. Thus, the cold is not so much a
disease as a syndrome, a collection of symptoms that often go together.

What we identify as colds are caused by upward of 150 different
viruses. Some of these are viruses that normally produce other, quite
different ailments, such as the MEASLES virus. Others, like the
adenoviruses, mostly cause more severe respiratory infections. But there
is one large group—a family of more than 100 closely related
members—that causes only colds and nothing else.

These last are the rhinoviruses (the name comes from a Greek word
meaning "nose," as in rhinoceros), and they must be considered the true
cold viruses. Since the true cause of most colds is never really pinned
down, nobody knows for sure what percentage of colds is caused by
rhinoviruses. They have been successfully found in from 25 to 30 percent
of the cases in which they have been sought. (And many of the failures are
probably due to the difficulties in growing the viruses rather than in their
absence.) In studies with volunteers living in isolation, dosage with
rhinoviruses regularly produces colds in 40 percent of the subjects.

The symptoms of a cold generally begin two to three days after
exposure, and the course of the disease can be divided into three stages.
Initially the victim is aware of an irritation, often a dryness, numbness, or
burning, in the nose or throat. Soon he is subject to a dry, sharp cough and
a feeling of heaviness or "stuffiness" about the nose and eyes. This is
accompanied by a headache, a sense of general discomfort, and in
children often a transient fever (which in an adult would be taken as a sign
of developing INFLUENZA). Most colds remain at this stage only a few
hours or at most a day or two. Some actually terminate at this point, and
the patient recovers without undergoing the full course.

Most commonly, on the second or third day the cold moves into its next, its acute phase. This stage is unmistakable: there is a profuse, watery, nasal discharge, and an almost constant need to "blow" the nose. At this point also the patient is subject to frequent sneezing and a heavier cough, which now produces mucus. Actually, the onset of this stage may bring some sense of relief, though the discharge itself seems an almost endless burden. The headache, malaise, tension about the nose and eyes, and any low-grade fever, all disappear, and at this point the cold is said to "break."

As this second stage persists, the discharge thickens, becomes yellowed, and is more difficult to release. Some measure of stuffiness and tension may then return, as the cold moves into its third phase, which often lasts about a week. Now, because of the thickening of the mucus, the nostrils may be obstructed, which can make breathing difficult, and the cough becomes heavy and rattling. Sometimes there is a persistent postnasal drip or a laryngitis. Gradually, however, following a somewhat uneven pattern, all the symptoms diminish and ultimately disappear.

The typical rhinovirus cold appears to be a superficial infection of the respiratory tract. The virus invades the mucous membranes of the nose and throat, multiplies, and provokes the local symptoms. Unlike most virus diseases, rhinovirus infection does not pass through a phase of heavy virus multiplication in the bloodstream. Such a stage of *viremia* is usually accompanied by high fever and really prostrating illness, both of which are usually missing with a cold. This localization of the infection is probably linked with a penchant of the virus for multiplying only at temperatures somewhat below normal body temperature, a condition that is found in the upper respiratory tract.

The way we catch colds is still not fully understood. It is clear enough that colds do spread from person to person. It is known that viruses are contained in nose and throat secretions, and that we send viruses out into the air with every cough and sneeze, that handkerchiefs and possibly pillows become heavily impregnated, and that we generally spread the virus all around our living space. But how others actually take in the viruses is still somewhat uncertain. The simplest assumption is that they inhale virus-laden droplets from the air. But in one study it was found that viruses were most easily picked up on the hands—from touching other persons' environmental surfaces—and then transported to the nose or eyes, where they entered the body through the mucous membranes.

Surprisingly, colds do not really seem to be very contagious. In other studies—of adult couples living together, one of whom was infected and one not—the virus spread to the partner in only 38 percent of the cases, in spite of as many as 17 hours a day spent in each other's company.

It is generally believed that the onset of colds is influenced by the weather and by the effects of fatigue and chilling (hence the name). It is true that, although colds occur at any time in the tropics, in more temperate areas they are largely a winter disease. No one knows quite why this should be (but many diseases show unexplained seasonal variations). One supposition is that mucous membranes dry out in the winter months from lack of humidity and thus are more susceptible to virus attack. (The use of humidifiers in winter seems to reduce the incidence of colds for many people.)

Whether or not chilling increases susceptibility to colds is still a matter of contention. A rash of colds often follows the first winter storms, but it has been suggested that it is the change in weather that is important, not the chilling effect of the cold. Fatigue and "lowered resistance," supposedly resulting from a lack of sleep, poor diet, and tension, may contribute to susceptibility, but the evidence is not conclusive on this score. Certainly one can keep warm in the winter, eat properly, get plenty of rest, and still catch a cold, but maybe if he does all these things he is a little less likely to catch one.

Also, there is the puzzling matter of individual differences in susceptibility—some people claim never to have colds at all; others seem to have far more than their share. Of course, very little is known about variation in susceptibility to diseases in general, and other diseases show similar effects. Still, with colds, the discrepancy seems more marked: in one study, a quarter of the participants had three quarters of the colds.

It is not clear to what extent colds leave immunity behind them. Superficially, the answer would seem to be "not much," since most people experience several colds in succession each year. But when one considers the number of different viruses that can cause colds, it becomes clear that each new cold could be an infection by a new and different virus. If there are 150 of these, one could have two colds a year over the average lifetime and still not have exhausted all the possibilities. The fact that children have more colds than adults could reflect the circumstance that they are less likely than adults to encounter cold viruses they have already been exposed to and have developed immunity against.

Some of the rather puzzling information about individual susceptibility to colds could be explained by immunity. In studies in which only a small percentage of the individuals exposed to a particular virus actually catch cold, it could be that the rest have already been exposed and are immune. In the 18th century, when a community still could be quite completely isolated from the rest of the world, the approach of a stranger would often bring colds to everyone in the community, not to just a susceptible few. Boswell in his "Life of Johnson" refers to a story reported by Macaulay that whenever a ship arrived at the isolated island of St. Kilda in the Hebrides, everyone caught cold. Boswell attributed this to the wind that brought the ship in; we would say that someone aboard the ship carried a cold virus to which no one had been exposed and against which no one had immunity.

The common cold is not the sort of disease that warrants elaborate diagnostic procedures—it is usually not life-threatening—and, in any case, the symptoms alone are unmistakable. But there are times when it may be necessary to determine that a cold is not simply a very mild form of some more serious disease, which could be a danger to others. For research purposes, too, it is sometimes desired to pinpoint precisely the cause of a cold. Under any such circumstances, virus isolation procedures are used. The best source of viruses is nasal secretions. These are mixed with various kinds of cells in *tissue cultures,* and characteristic changes in the cells signal the presence of rhinoviruses or other possible viruses. The exact identity of the virus is determined by tests with known *antibodies.* Once the virus has been identified, a rise in blood levels of antibodies to that virus may be sought to confirm that it is the cause of the infection.

The best treatment for a cold is to make the patient as comfortable as possible and let the cold run its course. The patient should keep warm and get plenty of rest. A hot, humid environment seems to ease the discomfort of the nose and throat; inhalation of steam may be helpful. Gargling with hot salt water is recommended. Although one frequently hears that drinking large amounts of liquids is good for colds, there seems to be little evidence for this belief—still, hot drinks do soothe the throat; hot lemonade, tea, even the proverbial chicken soup, may be helpful.

As for medication, throat lozenges and cough syrups, especially those containing codeine or other cough suppressants, also ease the throat. Drops containing vasoconstricting drugs (chemical agents that cause blood vessels to narrow) may be used to relieve the congestion of the nose. They should be used sparingly, however, for their initial effect is often followed by a "backlash" of increased flow of fluid. Aspirin and certain other analgesics are most useful in easing headaches, mitigating physical discomfort, reducing fever (if there is any), and permitting sleep. (Some researchers have found that aspirin increases the number of rhinoviruses shed by cold sufferers, but the risk of increasing the spread of the virus in this way is deemed so small, and the value of aspirin in relieving cold symptoms is so great, that authorities continue to recommend its use.)

Numerous cold medications containing different combinations of these kinds of ingredients—cough suppressants, nasal decongestants, and analgesics—are available without prescription. It must be emphasized that none of these products cures colds or even shortens their duration, but they may relieve the symptoms and make the patient more comfortable. There is no reason they should not be used, provided the directions are carefully followed and the use is not prolonged. At one time it was thought that antihistamines relieved cold symptoms, but careful trials seem to have disproved this contention (although antihistamines are effective against hay fever and other allergies).

The sheer multiplicity of cold remedies may be something of a problem; it is said that there are as many as 50,000 such products on the market. Can they all be equally effective? They are certainly "big business"—it is estimated that the American public spends three quarters of a billion dollars a year on them. Much of this sale results from extensive advertising, which must be carefully watched. None of these products can be said to cure; they can only be described as relieving symptoms.

In 1972 the National Academy of Sciences released a report prepared for the Food and Drug Administration on the effectiveness of 27 different over-the-counter cold remedies. Although a number were deemed useful against hay fever, only a handful were found at all effective even in relieving the symptoms of colds.

A more ambitious study of all nonprescription cold remedies was then carried out for the FDA by a government-sponsored panel of scientists. Reporting in September 1976, the panel concluded that most of the products contained too many ingredients, with many of them ineffective or present in too small amounts. Of the 120 most common ingredients, the panel found only 44 clearly safe and effective, with more research needed to establish the efficacy of most of the rest. (Some, it was recommended, should be removed.) On the panel's advice, the FDA agreed to release 10 drugs for over-the-counter use that had previously been permitted only in prescription drugs: 5 antihistamines, 2 bronchodilators, and 3 nasal decongestants. Finally, the panel recommended that all over-the-counter cold remedies contain no more than 3 active ingredients—one for nasal decongestion, one for cough, and one for headache.

As is true of other virus diseases, colds do not respond to ordinary antibiotics, and unless bacterial complications actually appear, the use of antibiotics is not advised. Contrary to this advice, however, many physicians routinely prescribe antibiotics for cold sufferers, supposedly either to forestall complications or on the ground that a mixed infection may already exist. This practice is discouraged because it can open the way to infection by antibiotic-resistant strains of bacteria, which then may be very difficult to eliminate.

The status of vitamin C as a cold preventive or cure, or both, remains problematic. About as many tests reporting favorable as unfavorable results exist, and though most responsible medical and nutritional experts feel that the vitamin is probably of little or no value, a persistent group of vitamin C proponents continues to argue for use of the vitamin. The best conclusion would seem to be that, for the present, the case for vitamin C remains unproved. A review of 30 years of research on vitamin C and colds, which was published in 1975 in the "Journal of the American Medical Association," faults most of the pro-vitamin C research and concludes that there is "little convincing evidence to support claims of clinically important efficacy."

One trouble with vitamin C as a cold remedy is that massive doses are called for—up to four to eight grams a day, 100 times the amount officially recommended for regular intake. And there is some evidence that such large amounts of the vitamin may themselves create medical problems, such as bleeding gums, circulatory disturbances, and the formation of kidney stones.

In fact, vitamin C is not the only vitamin that has been proposed as a cold preventive. Some people advocate the use of various of the B vitamins, especially folic acid. But here, too, the proposal is suspect.

In their search for drugs to fight viruses, scientists have uncovered several that show promise against rhinoviruses. One group has reported that a urea derivative* inhibits the growth of rhinoviruses. This drug has yet to undergo testing in human beings.

Another promising lead involves the substance propanediamine, which acts as an *interferon-inducer,* a material that causes the body cells to produce their own antiviral agent, interferon. When propanediamine nose drops were given to persons freshly exposed to rhinoviruses, most of those treated experienced far fewer colds than did control subjects exposed to the viruses but not given the drug. (Purified interferon from human subjects has been shown to be active against colds, but the substance is too expensive to be practical.)

Also, a new immunotherapeutic agent, a drug that stimulates the immunity system to fight off invading viruses, has been found effective

---

*The chemical name of the drug is N-*p*-chlorophenyl-N'-(*m*-isobutyl-guanidinophenyl)-urea hydrochloride.

against rhinoviruses. This drug, which is called inosiplex, is reported to produce significant reductions in frequency of colds and in their severity. Although none of the compounds that show promise against rhinoviruses in tests has yet come into use, it is hoped that before long a good anticold drug will be available, one which will not just ease the symptoms of a cold, but will actually cure or prevent it.

The preparation of cold vaccines is difficult—well nigh impossible—because there are so many different viruses that can cause colds that to immunize against all of them would be a horrendous task. It may turn out, however, that some rhinoviruses are more common than others, or cause more severe colds, and one could then immunize against these alone. Or it might be that there is some cross-immunity with rhinoviruses, that immunizing against a few of them would produce immunity against many others. (This seems unlikely, though, because natural immunity against rhinoviruses apparently does not act this way.)

Another problem is the superficial nature of the cold itself. A cold vaccine injected into the bloodstream might not produce antibodies in the limited area of the mucous membranes of the upper respiratory tract where the rhinoviruses operate. So, in fact, a cold vaccine might be effective only if sprayed into the nose and throat, where it could presumably produce a localized immunity. Naturally, the effectiveness of any cold vaccine would depend on the degree of immunity brought about by rhinoviruses—a matter, as indicated above, that is open to conjecture. Still, all thing considered, it is possible that someday nasal spray vaccines will be able to offer a degree of protection against at least certain common rhinoviruses.

The rhinoviruses are classed as picorna viruses—small ("pico" means, among other things, a small quantity in Spanish), *RNA*-containing viruses, about 30 nanometers (one millionth of an inch) in diameter. The particles are *icosahedral* and do not have an *outer envelope*. The hundred or so different rhinoviruses vary presumably only in minor surface details, which do not show up in the electron microscope. The different types can be distinguished by the antibodies they cause to be formed.

Rhinoviruses grow best under neutral conditions and at a temperature of about 91° F, considerably lower than body temperature, 98.6°. They much resemble the POLIO virus and other enteroviruses physically and in their behavior, but unlike the enteroviruses, they are easily destroyed by acid. For this reason, rhinoviruses do not survive passage through the stomach (though vast numbers of them may be swallowed when one has a cold), and again unlike enteroviruses, they are never found in the stools.

CONDYLOMAS. See WARTS.

CONNECTIVE TISSUE DISEASE (RHEUMATIC DISEASE, COL-LAGEN DISEASE). A number of diseases affect the connective tissue—that is, the supporting tissue of the various body organs and parts, which chiefly takes the form of cartilage, membranes, ligaments, and tendons. Often these diseases involve considerable pain—generally inflammation is an important element—and in extreme cases they can be severely crippling or otherwise disabling. Like ARTHRITIS, the best known of these diseases, most of them are chronic, persisting over the patient's lifetime, though of course there are acute, or transient, disorders of the connective tissues also. It is suspected that arthritis and another member of this family of diseases, SYSTEMIC LUPUS ERYTHE-MATOSUS, belong to the category of SLOW VIRUS DISEASE, and many authorities believe that ultimately all the chronic diseases of this type will be placed in that category.

In addition to arthritis and lupus, this group also includes gout, a metabolic disorder that causes uric acid crystals to be deposited in the joints, and ankylosing spondylitis, a disease of the spine, which leads to fusion of the vertebrae. Another connective tissue disease, rheumatic fever, which follows streptococcal infections (like "strep throat"), usually consists of an arthritislike disorder of the joints and an inflammation of the valves of the heart.

Other diseases often grouped with these are Sjogren's syndrome, which is characterized by a drying up of the tear ducts and the salivary glands; scleroderma, a thickening and hardening of the skin and certain of the internal organs; polyarteritis (or periarteritis nodosa), a generalized inflammation of the arterial walls; and dermatomyosis, an inflammatory process affecting the skin and muscle tissue.

Although these disorders are often called "connective tissue diseases," technically they are referred to as "rheumatic diseases," a general term for disorders of the muscles and joints. Sometimes, less commonly, they are classed as "collagen diseases," collagen being a protein that is an important component of connective tissue.

In spite of the chronic inflammation of connective tissue that these diseases all have in common, they may or may not be closely related. As to what causes them, this is still largely unknown. In many of them, however, there seems to be a combination of inherited tendency—some kind of a genetic predisposition—and a triggering infection, possibly viral.

COXSACKIE OR ECHO VIRUS INFECTION. Most infections caused by the coxsackie and echo viruses are *inapparent*—that is, not accompanied by noticeable symptoms. Nevertheless, the many viruses in these families are responsible for a number of ailments, ranging from mild colds to fatal heart disease. It is difficult to relate specific disorders to these viruses, however, for they produce a variety of respiratory, intestinal, cardiac, and neurological disturbances, most of which can also be caused by other viruses. In particular, they sometimes lead to a disease that is very much like POLIO, a fact that is not surprising since the coxsackie and echo viruses are physically almost indistinguishable from the polio virus. There are, to be sure, two disorders, HERPANGINA and epidemic PLEURODYNIA, attributed exclusively to coxsackie viruses, and in time more diseases are likely to be identified as due to viruses of both groups. No vaccines against these viruses have been prepared.

The first coxsackie virus was isolated in 1948 from two polio patients in the town of Coxsackie, N.Y. Because these patients were also infected with the polio virus, the role of the coxsackie virus in their disorder was uncertain. A few years later the first echo viruses were found—and named as an acronym for *e*nteric *c*ytopathic *h*uman *o*rphan, meaning that the viruses were (1) isolated from the enteric, or intestinal, tract; (2) destructive of cells in culture; (3) associated with the human body; and (4) not connected with any known disease.

Initially, these viruses were thought to be more or less harmless "passengers" that rode along with the body but did no appreciable damage. Now, however, of the 30 different viruses of each kind that have been found, most are associated with diseases of one sort or another. Nonetheless, it is still true that a large percentage of the persons infected with these viruses do not become ill at all. Although it is difficult to generalize, the coxsackie viruses as a group seem to cause serious illness more frequently that the echo viruses do. The latter are distinguished in the laboratory for their failure to produce ill effects in mice and hamsters.

The echo and coxsackie viruses, like the polio virus, are classed as enteroviruses because they multiply chiefly in the intestinal tract. Accordingly, it might be suspected that they would be likely to cause cases of "stomach flu," or *epidemic* GASTROENTERITIS, and indeed outbreaks of this disorder in young children in summer have been traced to echo viruses. Also, vomiting and other signs of upset stomach are often included in the symptoms produced by both echo and coxsackie viruses.

The most typical disorder associated with these viruses is a generalized feverish illness, often accompanied by a rash on various parts of the body. This is a generally mild, measleslike ailment of short duration—a few days to a week—and it usually goes undiagnosed or is characterized simply as a "virus" infection. Sometimes, however, certain special signs are present, and the resulting disorder is clearly recognized and given a name of its own. Herpangina, in which the rash is limited to the inside of the mouth, is one such disorder.

Another, similar disease is the so-called "hand, foot, and mouth disease," in which a rash appears within the mouth as well as on the palms of the hands and the soles of the feet. It is accompanied by a sore throat, coldlike symptoms, and abdominal pain, possibly diarrhea. Hand, foot, and mouth disease has been found to be caused by coxsackie virus A16, and at times by other coxsackie A viruses. (The coxsackie viruses are divided into A and B groups, according to the symptoms they produce in mice.)

A similar but milder disorder is the "Boston exanthema" (an exanthema being a disease accompanied by rash). The peculiar feature of this disorder is that the rash, which covers the face, chest, and back—sometimes the whole body—does not appear until the fever has subsided and other signs of illness have disappeared. The disease was first observed in Boston in 1951; it is produced by echo virus 16.

The point at which the echo and coxsackie viruses first multiply in the body is the nose and throat, and most disorders caused by these viruses show some signs of throat involvement—usually sore throat and cough. Furthermore, many conditions that would normally pass for THE COMMON COLD or INFLUENZA have been shown (by virus isolation) actually to have been caused by echo or coxsackie viruses. Undoubtedly many more such cases go undiagnosed.

Like the polio virus, the coxsackie and echo viruses have a penchant for nerve tissue, and cause disorders of the nervous system. Now that extensive use of polio vaccines has greatly reduced the incidence of true polio, more and more instances of poliolike disease caused by the echo and coxsackie viruses are coming to light. Since the first isolation of coxsackie viruses from patients also infected with polio virus, many more such instances of joint infection have been found, and when paralysis occurs, it is not really clear which virus is the major culprit. (Paradoxically, some echo and coxsackie viruses also interfere with infection by polio viruses and, when they are present at the time of vaccination, prevent the vaccination from taking.)

Actually, the number of cases of paralytic disease caused by echo and coxsackie viruses is small, but these viruses are responsible for many cases of nonparalytic "polio." Typically, these are feverish illnesses of week-long duration, accompanied by MENINGITIS or ENCEPHALITIS

—signaled by headache, stiff back and neck, possibly unusual drowsiness. Often echo virus meningitis is characterized by an attendant rash, and coxsackie virus meningitis by chest pains.

It now seems clear that coxsackie viruses (and, to a lesser extent, echo viruses) do have a tendency to attack the muscles and membranes of the chest and heart, with the result that chest pain is a frequent concomitant of coxsackie virus infection. Epidemic pleurodynia is a disorder in which this is the major sign.

The most serious disease in this category is myocarditis, inflammation of the heart muscle. Sometimes called Fiedler's myocarditis, this is a devastating disease of the newborn, which often leads to heart failure. The fatality rate in infants is about 50 percent. The disorder, known since the late 19th century, frequently occurs as epidemics in hospitals. Several such epidemics have been traced to single infants born of mothers who have had coxsackie virus infections. Some cases of myocarditis appear to be due to infection by coxsackie A viruses, and even echo viruses, and at times no virus can be found at all. Myocarditis also affects older children and adults, and here too, though the fatality rate is lower, the disease can be troublesome.

Pericarditis, inflammation of the membrane surrounding the heart, is also an occasional result of coxsackie B virus infection, sometimes also of A virus infection. It can occur along with pleurodynia. Though any involvement of the heart is a serious matter, pericarditis is less likely than myocarditis to cause major HEART DISEASE, or death.

Finally, certain of the coxsackie viruses seem to be associated with juvenile ARTHRITIS and possibly even DIABETES. In several instances coxsackie virus infection has been observed immediately before the appearance of arthritis symptoms in young persons, but proof of a causal connection between the two is lacking. In diabetes, the suspicion stems from the fact that several coxsackie viruses in mice damage the pancreas in much the way it is damaged in human diabetes.

Although the echo and coxsackie viruses are probably spread—like the polio virus—chiefly in fecal matter, they may also be emitted from the nose and throat, especially when there are coldlike symptoms. Children are the chief source of infection, and the viruses spread rapidly through schools and households with children. Echo and coxsackie viruses occur everywhere in the world, and they circulate most abundantly in the summer months when minor epidemics of the various ailments they cause appear. Most people, during their lifetime, are exposed to a number of these viruses even though they experience no major illness as a result.

Not much is known about the movement of coxsackie and echo viruses in the body, nor about how they cause particular symptoms. It seems that they must invade the body in the throat (or possibly the nose) and travel through the alimentary tract to multiply in the intestinal area. In time they must invade the bloodstream and, ultimately, the skin, the nervous system, the muscles and membranes of the chest and heart, or the mucous membranes of the mouth, nose, or throat. The particular area of the body that becomes the focus for virus attack determines the symptoms that are observed. Variable and not-yet-understood aspects of the virus's structure and the susceptibility or resistance of the various tissues of the human host must direct the attack.

There is no specific remedy for echo or coxsackie virus infection, no drug that kills the viruses. Thus, treatment is mostly palliative, limited to making the patient as comfortable as possible. Aspirin is the chief remedy used with the cold- and flu-like disorders. When encephalitis or meningitis is observed, a physician should be consulted. Myocarditis of the newborn is, of course, a serious matter, and if the infant is not still in the hospital he must be hospitalized.

Because there are so many varieties of coxsackie and echo viruses, the prospects of preparing vaccines against them is not good. But as more is learned about the different viruses, particular types may emerge as the most prevalent or the cause of the most serious ailments, and vaccines against them may then be prepared. In this connection, it is already known that there are only six coxsackie B viruses and that they are the chief cause of infant myocarditis—hence these might well be prime targets for vaccine development.

Since the echo and coxsackie viruses cause so many different illnesses, most of which are also produced by other agents, conclusive diagnosis must always be by laboratory methods—although, of course, with minor ailments, accurate diagnosis is not really necessary. The best source of viruses for purposes of identification is the stools, but viruses also may be found on throat swabs, in cerebrospinal fluid, or in matter drawn from skin or mouth sores. Coxsackie viruses are detected by the characteristic damage they cause newborn mice or hamsters or by the changes they produce in *cultured* cells; echo viruses, only by the latter changes. Identification of the specific virus present is by tests with *antibodies* against known viruses. Even when viruses are not isolated, the presence of infection can be confirmed by a sharp rise in antibodies to the virus in the blood during the course of the illness (such determinations usually being made by *serologic tests*).

The particles of the echo and coxsackie viruses are physically almost exactly alike, approximately spherical (*icosahedral*) and about 30 nanometers (one millionth of an inch) in diameter. The *nucleic acid*, which comprises about 30 percent of the particle, is single-stranded RNA. So far, some 30 different echo viruses have been identified, along with 24 coxsackie A viruses and the 6 B viruses.

CREUTZFELDT-JAKOB DISEASE. A rare and always fatal disorder of the brain, the Creutzfeldt-Jakob disease is one of the few human degenerative diseases rather clearly shown to be caused by a virus, or viruslike agent. Typical symptoms include forgetfulness, loss of coordination, blurring of vision, and spastic movements of the arms and legs. The ultimate outcome, after a period of some months or years, is coma and paralysis. The disease has been said to resemble PARKINSON'S DISEASE plus dementia, or complete loss of mental ability. Often mental activity has ceased completely before the inert patient dies of some other cause, usually pneumonia. Some authorities believe that the disease is not so rare as it seems—only about 200 cases have been reported in the medical literature—with many cases being simply diagnosed as presenile dementia, a catchall term. In fact, it has been suggested that there may be as many as several hundred deaths a year from the disease in the United States alone.

As revealed by autopsy, the immediate cause of the symptoms of Creutzfeldt-Jakob disease—the disorder, incidentally, is named after two of the first physicians to study it—is massive destruction of brain tissue. Nerve cells are almost completely eaten away, and the remaining brain matter has a spongy look when observed under the microscope. In this respect this disease much resembles KURU, a disorder experienced solely by a tribe of New Guinea cannibals, and two animal diseases, scrapie of sheep and transmissible mink encephalopathy.*

Like these disorders, the Creutzfeldt-Jakob disease is generally classed as a SLOW VIRUS DISEASE, though the evidence that a virus is involved is somewhat indirect. To begin with, these diseases are infectious—Creutzfeldt-Jakob disease can be transmitted to chimpanzees, guinea pigs, and mice by injection of infected brain material from human beings. And scientists have failed to find any signs of bacteria or other cellular organisms in such material, usually a clear indication that a virus is involved. But no viruses can be seen in electron micrographs—all that is observed is unusual, curled bits of cell membrane. In other respects

---

*In certain ways, also, several more common degenerative nervous-system diseases—namely, Alzheimer's disease, Huntington's chorea, and Peck's disease—are similar to these.

too this agent is unusual: it is extremely resistant to agents that inactivate most viruses, including formaldehyde and ultraviolet radiation; it does not cause the usual *antibodies* to form in the bodies of its victims; and it is smaller than any known virus. Some authorities speculate that the agent of these diseases is actually a bit of aberrant cell membrane; others, that it is a new kind of microorganism altogether.

It is not known how the "virus" of Creutzfeldt-Jakob disease is transmitted in nature. In certain areas of the world the disease is more prevalent, and many signs suggest that it has a hereditary aspect (as seems also to be the case with kuru). But the disease apparently can be transmitted (again, like kuru) by the consumption or handling of infected brain matter. A recent outbreak among Libyan Jews living in Israel has been tentatively traced to a Libyan habit of eating sheep and cattle brains. And in the case of a neurosurgeon who died of the disease, it is suspected that he may have acquired it through contact with infected brain material.

In another bizarre and tragic circumstance, a patient was inadvertently given corneal transplants from a person later shown to have died of Creutzfeldt-Jakob disease. Within two years the transplant patient too had died of the disease, an event—considering the rarity of the disease—unlikely to be coincidental.

These happenings suggest certain warnings for those handling neurological materials and those selecting donors for transplants, but they do not shed light on how the agent of Creutzfeldt-Jakob disease is transmitted under more usual circumstances. Like the nature of the agent itself, this remains something of a medical mystery.

CRIB DEATH. See SUDDEN INFANT DEATH SYNDROME.

CRIMEAN HEMORRHAGIC FEVER. See HEMORRHAGIC FEVER.

CROHN'S DISEASE (REGIONAL ENTERITIS, REGIONAL ILEITIS) AND ULCERATIVE COLITIS. Chronic diseases of the upper and lower bowel, respectively, Crohn's disease and ulcerative colitis both are characterized by abdominal pain, often severe; chronic diarrhea, sometimes with bloody discharges; and extended fever, anemia, weakness, and weight loss. Evidence is accumulating that both diseases are virus-caused (possibly by the same agent), and it is likely that they fall into the general category of SLOW VIRUS DISEASE.

First described in 1932 by the American physician Burill Crohn, Crohn's disease is an inflammatory disorder of the ileum, the lower end of the small intestine. (It is also referred to as regional enteritis or regional ileitis.) Although Crohn's disease hits people of all ages it is found most frequently in two groups: the young, between the ages of 15 and 30, and those just past middle age, from 50 to 60. The disease is of growing importance; in 1977 it was estimated that 70 to 80 of every 100,000 Americans had the disease—a figure that had more than doubled in two years.

Ulcerative colitis, which has been known much longer (since 1895), affects the colon, the lower, or large, bowel. It strikes most commonly those aged 20 to 40, and its incidence too is rising.

Although both diseases have been known to occur in brief, acute episodes, followed by complete recovery, a slow, progressive course, with temporary or partial improvement, followed by recurrences and relapses, is more common. Some patients are chronically ill for many years. Ulcers and perforations of the intestinal wall are serious aspects of the disease. Secondary bacterial infections are the most common complication; cancer of the ileum or colon are the most serious.

In mild cases, bed rest and a bland diet may provide sufficient therapy to bring the disease under control. Intravenous feeding, to avoid the digestive tract, is sometimes resorted to, and steroids and other anti-inflammatory drugs are often used. In extreme cases, surgery to remove small or large segments of the bowel may become necessary.

Evidence that these diseases are caused by one or more viruses is of two types. Neither by itself is conclusive, but taken together they are quite suggestive.

The first line of evidence is that bowel tissue taken from patients with both diseases can transmit the disease to mice and rabbits. The active agent in this tissue is of virus size (as shown by its ability to pass through fine filters), and it is destroyed by heat and phenol treatment, as would be expected of a virus. Whereas mice responded similarly to the tissues from Crohn's disease patients and from those with ulcerative colitis, the rabbits responded differently, suggesting—though not proving—that the agents in the two tissues are not the same.

The second line of evidence involves the viruslike cell-destroying activity of tissue from patients with these diseases when tested against human cell cultures. The agent responsible for this action is thought to be a small RNA virus, which is found in patients with a number of intestinal disorders, in addition to those discussed here. It may be identical with a particle observed by the electron microscope in Crohn's disease patients, but not others. This particle is described as 30 nanometers in diameter (about one millionth of an inch), and resembling a picornavirus, the family of small RNA viruses that the POLIO, echo, and coxsackie viruses belong to (see COXSACKIE OR ECHO VIRUS INFECTION). Significantly, perhaps, all these viruses are known to inhabit the human intestinal tract.

CROUP. See RESPIRATORY INFECTION.

CYTOMEGALIC INCLUSION DISEASE. See CYTOMEGALOVIRUS INFECTION.

CYTOMEGALOVIRUS INFECTION. Virtually unknown to the general public, cytomegalovirus infection is a major cause of birth defects and premature death in infants. Some 4,000 children a year in the United States alone are born with mental retardation because of this disorder. Cytomegalovirus infection also causes blindness, deafness, and often fatal damage to the internal organs. In all, it is a more serious threat to the newborn than GERMAN MEASLES. Like that disease, cytomegalovirus infection is acquired from the mother, but the problem is especially insidious because the mother herself experiences no ill effects and does not know of the infection. Under special circumstances, cytomegalovirus does cause a form of MONONUCLEOSIS in adults, and perhaps certain other disorders. At present there is no specific drug or vaccine to be used against the virus, but experimental work in both areas is encouraging.

The cytomegalovirus gets its name from peculiar, large cells ("cyto-," cell; "mega-," large) that were first observed in the internal organs of stillborn infants in the early 1900s. At first these cells were thought to be parasites, but it was soon realized that they were human cells that had been altered in some way so that they contained dark areas called "inclusions" or "inclusion bodies." Shortly afterward, the same kinds of cells were found in the salivary glands of guinea pigs and other animals, and in 1926 it was shown that in guinea pigs these cells were produced by a virus. By 1950 it was quite well established that the inclusion-bearing cells were associated with a distinct disease in newborn children, a disease variously called "salivary gland virus infection," "inclusion body disease," and—the name preferred today—"cytomegalic inclusion disease." In 1956 the cytomegalovirus that infects human beings was discovered.

Today we know that many more newborn children are infected with this virus than show signs of disease—it is estimated that one percent of all children born are infected, but that only 10 percent of these actually suffer from the cytomegalic inclusion disease. (In the symptomless cases, the virus can be detected even though the symptoms do not appear.) When the disease is present, many of the symptoms show up at birth or within 48 hours afterward. These include jaundice, pneumonia, blindness, deafness, enlargement of the spleen and liver, small-head formation (microcephaly), a dark reddening of the skin (purpura), and internal bleeding. Frequently a child is born prematurely and is underweight. As indicated at autopsy, many cases of spontaneous abortion and stillbirth result from this disorder. Usually the condition of the newborn child with cytomegalic inclusion disease worsens steadily, and death may result within a matter of weeks. Many survive, however, and are permanently impaired, physically or mentally. Several of the symptoms, including mental retardation and deafness, may not be detected for some months, and at times these appear even when the other symptoms are not present. Some authorities believe that the virus takes a heavier toll in this respect than is commonly realized.

There are two schools of thought regarding transmission of the virus from the mother to the child. One school holds that the virus must be present in the mother's blood during the early stages of pregnancy—possibly in the first three months, as is the case with the German measles virus—and that the virus moves with the maternal blood through the placenta to the fetus. In support of this position is the fact that many victims of the disease show abnormalities of a kind that suggest the virus has interfered with their development rather than caused damage after development was already completed, though this is not always easy to determine.

According to the other school, the virus is actually transferred to the child only during birth—it is present in the cervix, and the infant encounters it as he is being born, a process that is known to occur with the related HERPES virus. Supporting this thesis is the fact that it is often difficult to locate viruses in the mother's blood, but usually easy to find them in the cervix. Probably both schools are right: it seems likely that infection of the fetus early in its development can occur, and that this accounts for the cases of complete cytomegalic inclusion disease with major defects. At the same time, infection during birth may also be possible, and this could explain the many instances of infection with only minor disease or with no apparent symptoms at all. Also, it cannot be excluded that infected infants spread the virus to other children (or to their adult handlers) early in the postnatal period.

Another open question is whether the maternal infections observed during pregnancy represent fresh invasions by the virus or reactivation of latent infections that have lain dormant for some time. Because many of these attacks seem limited to the cervical or urinary tract, it is suspected that they are recurrences of old infections, much as "cold sores" are repeating, localized outbreaks of herpes virus infection. It is known that herpes outbreaks can be stimulated by hormonal changes, and conceivably the hormonal changes of pregnancy could trigger cytomegalovirus recurrence. Possibly cytomegalovirus infection in women takes two forms: initial bodywide attacks (which, as indicated above, may affect the fetus early in its development), and repeating localized cervical infections, which occur during pregnancy and which spread to the child only at birth.

Yet, this repeating pattern has not definitely been established, and it is possible that the observed cervical infections are simply a late manifestation of the overall process—that the disease has passed through a stage of *viremia* and generalized infection and then centered in the cervical area. Also, it cannot be excluded that the localized infections are in fact limited, but result from venereal contact—researchers have found cytomegaloviruses in the semen of apparently healthy men—whereas more generalized infections come from some other mode of contact.

The virus is clearly widespread: *antibody* screening programs suggest that up to 80 percent of the population at large is exposed to the virus at one time or another. Undoubtedly, then, the virus is spread in ways not yet clearly established. Young children appear to be the most heavily infected, and even those with *inapparent infections* may shed viruses for several months in the urine, saliva, and other body secretions. Direct physical contact with infected persons appears to be necessary—the virus is fragile and does not survive long outside the body—and it is possible that the virus is taken into the body through the mouth, as well as in the ways already mentioned. It can also be spread by blood transfusion and organ transplantation. Young adults frequently harbor the virus, and it is not clear whether this is because they are likely to handle young children or because they are sexually active. The percentage of infected individuals is higher in lower socioeconomic groups and is especially high in underdeveloped countries. It seems safe to generalize that large families and poor personal hygiene contribute to spread of the virus.

Although most cytomegalovirus infections in older children and adults are inapparent, the virus can cause serious disease in older subjects, especially when the body defense mechanisms are impaired. This may be the case during debilitating illness such as CANCER, during extended steroid therapy, or during treatment with immunity suppressing drugs (following organ transplantation). In such situations the ailment resembles cytomegalic inclusion disease in infants, but it is likely to be limited to one or two organ systems—the liver, spleen, lungs, or intestinal tract. In individuals who have undergone multiple blood transfusions, as in open heart surgery, cytomegalovirus infection is likely to take the form of mononucleosis. Sometimes, peculiarly, this cytomegalovirus mononucleosis appears in persons who have had no blood transfusions at all.

On occasion, the cytomegalovirus attacks the central nervous system. Such attack represents an important aspect of cytoplasmic inclusion disease. But this virus has also been implicated in several cases of GUILLAIN-BARRÉ SYNDROME, a little understood, central nervous system disorder characterized by temporary paralysis. A clear connection between the virus and the disease has not definitely been established, however.

Finally, speculatively, it has been suggested that the cytomegalovirus may be involved in cases of human cancer. It has been observed that the cytomegalovirus is able to transform cells in *tissue culture* into a cancerlike form. Such experiments have been carried out with animal cells and also with human cells, but they are only suggestive—there is no proven connection between the cytomegalovirus and cancer. (Such a connection, if established, would be especially troublesome because of the widespread nature of the virus and the possibility that it is spread venereally.)

Treatment of cytomegalic inclusion disease in infants is difficult. Ordinary antibiotics and drugs have no effect on the virus, but several drugs now used against herpes viruses under special circumstances— idoxuridine, for example—also attack the cytomegalovirus. Unfortunately, such drugs are too toxic for bodywide use, as would be needed in combating cytomegalic inclusion disease. Much research is now being conducted on drugs that would be less toxic, and one new drug, still experimental, called phosphonoacetic acid, looks especially promising in animal tests.

Until such drugs are perfected, however, physicians have to rely on standard methods in treating children born with cytomegalic inclusion disease. The most immediate problem is blood loss due to hemorrhaging. Here multiple blood transfusions are called for; often the infant's entire blood supply must be replaced repeatedly. Constant provision of fluids intravenously also may be necessary. Although their use is sometimes questioned, steroids may be given in certain cases; antibiotics are employed only when there are secondary infections. Organ damage by the virus is the major permanent result of the disease, and often this is simply irremediable. In adult cases of cytomegalic inclusion disease, the situation is similar, though generally not so severe; treatment is likely to be simply palliative. With mononucleosis and the Guillain-Barré syndrome, complete bed rest is the chief therapy.

Several experimental *live-virus vaccines* against cytomegalovirus have been prepared. These are reported to produce antibodies in those vaccinated without causing serious side effects—though so many natural infections with this virus are inapparent, it may be difficult to prove that any attenuated virus is truly incapable of causing serious disease. The hope, of course, is to vaccinate young women before pregnancy, thereby preventing their becoming infected and passing the virus on to a child. There are several problems with this approach, however. One is establishing that the vaccine viruses do not remain in the mother's body and themselves reemerge at pregnancy to infect the developing fetus.

Another problem is reinfection. It is not at all clear that reinfection does not occur naturally with this virus, and if it does, vaccination could hardly be expected to prevent reinfection (since even a regular infection does not do so). In fact, the natural occurrence of repeating infections would suggest that antibodies caused by vaccine viruses might be unable to prevent reinfection by *wild viruses*.

Yet another drawback to widespread use of cytomegalovirus vaccines is the still unproven suspicion that the virus may be implicated in cancer. If so, introducing even weakened versions of the virus into the body as a vaccine might be unwise. Nevertheless, in spite of these various dangers, the damage caused to infants by cytomegalic inclusion disease is so great that efforts to develop a safe and effective method of vaccinating against it are obviously well spent.

Diagnosis of cytomegalovirus infection is almost always by laboratory procedures. The symptoms of cytomegalic inclusion disease in infants, while often distinctive, may sometimes be confused with those of other *congenital infections,* such as German measles. Often the disease is diagnosed in the laboratory by detection of the large, inclusion-containing cells that characterize the disease. These are found in urine specimens or tissue samples drawn from internal organs by biopsy and, after suitable staining, observed microscopically. Many times such cells occur in infants and adults who show no sign of disease.

Actual isolation of the causative virus is the best indication of cytomegalovirus infection. For this purpose urine specimens and throat swabs are taken. (In performing postmortem determinations on infants who have died presumably of cytomegalic inclusion disease, samples of tissue are used as the source of viruses.) The samples are mixed with cultures of human cells, and these are then watched for several days (or weeks in some cases) for the characteristic changes that signal the presence of cytomegalovirus.

In its structure, the cytomegalovirus resembles the herpes virus. The virus particles are large—about 110 nanometers (four millionths of an inch) in diameter—and surrounded by a double *outer membrane*. Within the nuclei of cells, where the virus particles form, they have only the inner membrane; the outer is acquired as the virus moves through the nuclear membrane into the body of the cell. The particle contains *DNA*, enclosed in a protein shell of *icosahedral* structure and composed of 162 well-defined protein subunits, all within the membranes.

As determined by experiments with antibodies, a number of strains of the virus exist, but how different they are and whether or not they deserve being called separate "types" is not yet certain. A whole series of closely related viruses has been found in the various animal species—mice, hamsters, monkeys, pigs, dogs, and so on—each species having its own virus, and each virus showing little or no ability to infect the cells of species other than its normal host. Human cytomegalovirus, therefore, cannot be cultivated in experimental animals; it is conveniently grown only in cultured human cells.

DANDY FEVER. See DENGUE.

DENGUE (DENGUE FEVER, BREAKBONE FEVER, DANDY FEVER). An infectious tropical and semitropical disease carried by mosquitoes, dengue is a serious, prostrating disorder but, under normal circumstances, rarely fatal. The principal symptoms are a high fever, acute joint aches, and a heavy rash. Bleeding from the nose and mouth is a fairly common occurrence, and in a second, often fatal, form of the disease, which is common among children in the Orient, hemorrhaging becomes the major symptom (see also HEMORRHAGIC FEVER). Although there is a true dengue virus that is responsible for most cases of the disease, dengue is actually a complex of virtually indistinguishable diseases caused by several different arboviruses (see ARBOVIRUS DISEASE).

Dengue has undoubtedly been around for a long time, but it was first described thoroughly in 1789 in Philadelphia by the pioneering American physician (and signer of the Declaration of Independence) Benjamin Rush, who gave it the name "bilious remitting fever." Because of the severe pain it causes in the joints, it was more commonly known in the

Americas as "breakbone fever." An alternate name, "dandy fever," is said by some authorities to be derived from the peculiar gait found in sufferers from the disease. More likely, however, this is a corruption of the old Spanish name for the disease, now the currently accepted name, dengue (pronounced DEN-gee or DEN-gay), which is said to be derived from an African word meaning fever.

Today dengue is *endemic* in large areas of the tropics, and *epidemics* occur periodically in the tropical and subtropical areas of virtually all continents. Southeast Asia and the Caribbean are favorite spots for epidemics; in 1969 some 17,000 cases occurred in Puerto Rico alone.

The virus nature of dengue was established in 1907, but it was not until 1944 that the dengue virus was actually isolated—from an American serviceman in Hawaii who was sick with the disease. Since then the virus has been detected in many parts of Asia and the Caribbean. In the 1950s four other viruses were isolated from patients with dengue or a denguelike ailment—chikungunya, o'nyong-nyong, and West Nile viruses in Africa and Mayaro virus in Trinidad. (Actually, West Nile virus had been isolated earlier but not from a dengue patient.) "Chikungunya" and "o'nyong-nyong" are native words meaning "doubling over," referring to the joint pain caused by the disease, and "Mayaro," like "West Nile," is the locality where the virus was first found, in this case a county on the island of Trinidad.

O'nyong-nyong virus is essentially limited to East Africa, but West Nile virus has caused outbreaks of dengue in much of West Africa, the Middle East, and India. Chikungunya virus was first found in Tanzania, but has since showed up in many parts of southern Africa and Southeast Asia. In Thailand and India it has been responsible for epidemics of the hemorrhagic form of dengue, both alone and in conjunction with the true dengue virus. Mayaro virus has been found only in Trinidad and Brazil.

It has been known since 1906 that dengue is transmitted by the bite of the mosquito. The chikungunya and true dengue viruses are carried by Aedes aegypti, which is also the *vector* of malaria and YELLOW FEVER. This species is a camp follower of man and chiefly inhabits towns and villages. The mosquito acquires the virus by biting an infected man, who carries the virus in his blood; then, after a period of 8 to 10 days during which the virus multiplies in the mosquito, the mosquito itself becomes infective and passes the virus on to each new person it bites.

In the laboratory, monkeys and mice can be infected with the dengue virus, and the detection of *antibodies* to the virus in wild animals in various parts of the world suggests that there are other animal hosts for the virus than man. These other animals are, most likely, infected by mosquitoes other than A. aegypti, whose chief victim is man. Nonetheless, true dengue and, probably, chikungunya fever remain essentially human diseases, with the virus passing mainly from man to man via the mosquito.

Not so with West Nile and Mayaro fever. Here the chief hosts for the virus are wild animals—monkeys in the case of Mayaro virus and wild birds with West Nile virus. Normally these viruses are spread from one wild animal to another by mosquitoes, and only occasionally is man infected. It is probably significant that these viruses are carried by mosquitoes other than A. aegypti, mosquitoes that feed chiefly on animal hosts—but sometimes on man.

The symptoms of dengue begin abruptly—after an *incubation period* of one week, give or take a few days. Chills, fever, intense headache, often localized directly behind the eyes, and excruciating backache and joint pains are the first signs. These generally persist for four to seven days, during which time the patient's face becomes red and puffy and he develops a light rash. Usually he is prostrate with the pain and fever. By this time his lymph glands are swollen, and blood tests reveal low white-cell counts.

In most cases, then, the fever breaks, with the patient washed in sweat, experiencing diarrhea and possibly bleeding from the nose and gums, but feeling suddenly, almost miraculously, better. About two-thirds of the time, however, this is short-lived: in a day or two the fever returns, and a heavy rash, characterized by small points of bleeding in the skin, spreads over the entire body. This persists for two or three days, and marks a period in which the patient is likely to be deeply depressed. Finally the rash begins to fade, with considerable itching and sloughing off of dead skin. Convalescence is slow—the patient is weak, unable to sleep, and subject to joint pains for some months. Recovery, however, is eventually complete.

No truly distinguishing features distinguish the dengue-like illnesses from true dengue. Often, though, they are reported as milder; West Nile fever, for example, is usually over quickly, and the hemorrhagic signs do not appear; but in epidemics it has been taken for true dengue.

In spite of the serious nature of dengue, death rates are generally low—less than one tenth of one percent. Experimental infection of volunteers shows that many cases of a mild, feverish dengue without great pain and with no rash also occur. These are present in any epidemic, and represent the prevailing pattern of illness in areas where the disease is endemic.

For reasons that are not clear, dengue complicated by severe hemorrhagic symptoms has been most common in Southeast Asia, where it primarily hits young children (while the adult population experiences the more normal disease). Some patients with hemorrhagic dengue have turned out to be simultaneously infected with chikungunya and dengue viruses, but either virus alone can cause this form of the disease.

After the dengue virus (or one of the other viruses described here) is inserted into the bloodstream by the bite of a mosquito, it multiplies extensively and travels to all parts of the body. It causes extensive damage in the walls of the smallest blood vessels everywhere, and is especially destructive of the softer tissues of the internal organs, such as the liver and the brain. The initial stage of major illness corresponds to the massive virus attack on the body tissues; the secondary attack, with heavy rash, seems to be an allergic response on the part of the body to the products of earlier cell damage by the virus.

There is no cure for dengue. The only treatment is to make the patient as comfortable as possible while the disease runs its course. Usually he is so ill that complete bed rest is mandatory. Except in very mild cases, hospitalization is advisable.

Although experimental *killed-virus vaccines* have failed to give protection against the dengue virus, *live-virus vaccines* have been reported to be promising. The prospect of developing effective vaccines is somewhat clouded, however, by the fact that there are four types of the true dengue virus (and possibly more), as well as chikungunya and the other viruses involved in denguelike disease, and infection with any one of these does not give immunity against the others. Hence any vaccine would have to include complements of all these viruses to offer complete protection, a somewhat difficult assignment.

In the absence of a vaccine, the only method of controlling the disease is mosquito eradication. Since the outlawing of DDT and certain other insecticides, this is best accomplished by cleaning out mosquito breeding areas near human habitations. A. aegypti likes to breed in still pools of clean water, and uncovered village wells, cisterns, and jars of water are ideal for its use. Where forest dwelling mosquitoes are involved, the breeding areas may be more elusive. In the temperate zone, mosquito breeding and, consequently, dengue end with the first frost. In the tropics, both continue the year round.

Diagnosis of dengue is usually made easily on the basis of the sudden onset of the disease and the peculiar combinations of symptoms. Nevertheless, it is sometimes difficult to distinguish the disease from SANDFLY FEVER, yellow fever, and MEASLES, or any of a number of nonviral diseases, including malaria.

Laboratory diagnosis is almost always clear-cut, however. Any of the viruses causing dengue can be detected by injection of blood into the brains of newborn or suckling white mice, which then undergo EN-CEPHALITIS. Also, when blood containing any of these viruses is added to *tissue cultures,* the cells show characteristic changes. (Tissue samples of the internal organs, taken by biopsy·or at autopsy, also show the presence of the virus; but, peculiarly, viruses have been difficult to find in tissues from patients with the more severe hemorrhagic dengue.) To identify the virus involved, including the type of dengue virus, tests with known antibodies are performed. Finally, blood tests made early and late in the course of the illness show (by *serologic tests*) a sharp rise in antibodies to one of the viruses, and this too permits identification.

All the viruses involved in dengue are classed as arboviruses. Technically, the dengue and West Nile viruses belong to the group B arboviruses, whereas the chikungunya, o'nyong-nyong, and Mayaro viruses are in group A. The dengue and West Nile viruses are somewhat related to the viruses of yellow fever and Japanese encephalitis.

The particles of the dengue and West Nile viruses are small—variously reported as anywhere from 20 to 60 nanometers in diameter, with 40 nanometers (about a millionth of an inch) a good average. Roughly spherical (*icosahedral*), the particles are surrounded by an *outer membrane,* which seems to be quite easily deformed. They contain *RNA*. The other viruses, which have been less well studied, give every indication of having very similar structures.

DERMATOMYOSIS. See CONNECTIVE TISSUE DISEASE.

DEVIL'S GRIP. See PLEURODYNIA.

DIABETES (DIABETES MELLITUS, SUGAR DIABETES). A rather common metabolic disturbance, which results in the body's failure to utilize sugar properly, diabetes is characterized by excessive hunger and thirst, by weakness and easy fatigue, and by a tendency to pass copious amounts of urine. It is caused by a lack of the hormone insulin, and can be controlled by giving insulin by daily injection. Oral antidiabetic agents are not true substitutes for insulin, but in many patients they provide adequate control. Without treatment, the outcome is often diabetic coma and eventual early death. Even with treatment, diabetics are subject to many complications; as a result diabetes is the fifth-ranked cause of death by disease in the United States. It seems likely that a tendency to develop the disease in inherited, but there is some evidence that the malady itself is triggered by a virus infection. Many candidate viruses have been proposed, most often the MUMPS virus, but proof of a connection is still lacking.

Undoubtedly diabetes is a very old disease. It is described in writings from ancient Egypt, China, and India. The Greeks gave it its present name from a word meaning siphon, a reference to the abundant discharge of urine. The terms "sugar diabetes" and "diabetes mellitus" are later coinages reflecting the sugar content of diabetic urine (mellitus is from a Latin word for honey).

The relationship between diabetes and disturbance of the pancreas was first noticed by a British physician, Thomas Cawley, in 1778. By the early 20th century it was realized that diabetes was connected with destruction of small bodies of tissue embedded in the pancreas and called, after their discoverer, a 19th-century German physician, the "islets of Langerhans." It was concluded that these bodies produced a hormone, which was given the name insulin, from the Latin "insula," or island. In 1921 this hormone was isolated by Sir Frederick Banting and Charles H. Best, working in the Toronto Laboratory of J. J. R. Macleod. With perhaps some injustice, the Nobel Prize in Medicine in 1923 was awarded to Macleod and Banting, but not Best. (Banting shared his half of the award money with his coworker.)

Diabetes is a large and growing health problem. From 1950 to 1975 the estimated number of diabetics in the United States increased from 1.2 million to 5 million. (According to another estimate, the figure today is 10 million.) Although there is a form of juvenile diabetes, the typical victim is past the age of 40. Women are attacked slightly more frequently than men, and one quarter of all diabetics have relatives who also are diabetic. Overweight persons are more likely to develop the disease than those of normal weight, but it is not clear to what extent this is cause and to what extent effect.

Except in the young, whose initial attacks may be acute, diabetes begins slowly, and persons with mild cases may have the disease for a long time and not know it. The early, mild diabetic may experience unusual hunger, thirst, and weakness and may pass large amounts of urine, but more often than not what reveals the condition is the detection of sugar in the urine on routine physical examination. High levels of blood sugar under certain conditions are another sign that may appear on physical examination. In more severe cases, the so-called ketone bodies, such as acetone, make their appearance in the blood and urine. These substances are indirectly responsible for the condition of acidosis— excess acidity of the body—which is what causes diabetic coma.

It is well established that the failure of diabetics to produce sufficient insulin in the pancreas causes sugar not to be burned as it normally is, but to be excreted. To gain energy, then, the body oxidizes fat, and in the process produces an excess of the ketone bodies, which are at least partly responsible for the symptoms of the disease. .

Diabetes causes an unusual susceptibility to infection, and there are many complications. Minor skin infections occur, and resist treatment; gangrene may set in and cause the loss of toes, even the feet. Tuberculosis frequently develops. Influenza is a threat. Digestive troubles, kidney disorders, and HEART DISEASE are common. Vision may be impaired—even with insulin and other treatments available, diabetes is the second most important cause of blindness today.

But the most directly life-threatening effect is diabetic coma. This usually begins with a loss of appetite, a drop-off of the output of urine, and either diarrhea or constipation. Soon the patient collapses, and his breathing becomes labored; the breath and skin both acquire a peculiar, sweetish odor. In time the coma becomes complete, and death follows rapidly. Although this process once marked the leading cause of death among diabetics, today—with better treatment—death from diabetic coma is virtually unheard of; most deaths actually result from one or more complications.

The first successful treatment of diabetes consisted of diet control—the limitation of sugar intake. Mild cases today are still controlled in this way: it is estimated that more than half the diabetes patients receiving regular care require only diet therapy. But the discovery of insulin and the finding that insulin from animal sources (beef pancreas, for instance) could be given to human beings brought a new day to the treatment of more severe diabetes.

The daily injections of insulin—necessitated because the hormone would be broken down by the digestive enzymes if taken by mouth—are usually given before breakfast, at a dosage level carefully determined to keep the blood sugar at a near normal level. With proper attention to dosage level, and control of dietary sugar, even severe diabetics today can lead relatively normal lives. The life expectancy of most carefully treated patients is not far from that of the general population. To be sure, there is still danger from diabetic coma if the patient overindulges in sugar, but this can be stopped with prompt insulin injection. At the other extreme, overdosage of insulin or failure to consume the expected amounts of food leads to the condition described as insulin shock, the symptoms of which are hunger, fatigue, racing pulse, and pallor or flushing of the face, followed quickly by tremors, emotional upset, physical collapse, and unconsciousness. Rapid consumption of sugar halts the process almost immediately.

Because of the inconvenience and risk of infection associated with constant injections of insulin, investigators have developed several orally administered drugs to replace it, the first and best known of which is tolbutamine. These drugs are thought to act by stimulating the pancreas to produce more insulin; hence, they can be used only by patients already producing some of that hormone. Now, about equal numbers of patients are on insulin and on the oral agents.*

Although diabetes is being managed rather well today, medical investigators would like to develop new techniques that would do even better. Some authorities hold that a second hormone, glucagon, is also involved in diabetes, and if so, control of it as well as insulin might be expected to achieve better results. Also, experiments are being conducted on the transplantation of an intact pancreas, isolated islets of Langerhans, and even cultured cells derived from the islets. And work is being done on making an artificial pancreas, which could substitute in the body for the real thing.

Complete success in controlling diabetes is likely to come only when authorities know what causes it—and this is still largely a mystery. The role of viruses in the process—if any—is still unsettled. The first suggestion that diabetes might be due to a virus infection was made by a Norwegian physician in 1864—before viruses had even been discovered. He observed that one of his patients had developed diabetes following a mumps infection, and hypothesized a connection between the two.

Actually, there is now considerable epidemiological evidence linking viruses and juvenile diabetes. One study in New York State found that over a 25-year period mumps underwent a 7-year high/low cycle, which was closely reflected 4 years later by a juvenile diabetes cycle. Other evidence suggests that juvenile diabetes is present in an unexpectedly large number of children with congenital GERMAN MEASLES infections. And still other evidence—namely, the presence of *antibodies* to the virus in a high percentage of juvenile diabetics—implicates one of the coxsackie viruses (see COXSACKIE OR ECHO VIRUS INFECTION). Other viruses too have been tentatively included here—the HEPATITIS

---

*One oral antidiabetes drug, phenformin, was banned by the U.S. Department of Health, Education, and Welfare in July 1977 as an "imminent hazard to the public health." It had been implicated in more than 100 deaths resulting from acidosis.

and INFLUENZA viruses, as well as certain adeno-, entero-, and cyto-megaloviruses (see RESPIRATORY INFECTION and CYTOME-GALOVIRUS INFECTION).

Whatever the role of viruses in causing juvenile diabetes, it seems likely that there is a genetic predisposition involved—that some children are simply more susceptible than others to this malady. With diabetes that occurs in later life, there is much less evidence of a virus cause, and much clearer indication of a genetic role. If one identical twin, for example, becomes diabetic before the age of 40, there is a 50 percent chance the other will also; but if the first twin becomes diabetic after the age of 40, there is a 90 percent chance the other will.

There is some evidence that the inherited predisposition to diabetes may consist of a defect in the body's immunity system. This would place the disorder among the so-called autoimmune diseases, in which the immunity system is directed against some of the body's own cells—in this case the islet cells of the pancreas. In turn, this suggests that diabetes may be a type of SLOW VIRUS DISEASE, many others of which also seem to involve autoimmunity.

Much of the evidence linking diabetes in general with viruses comes from animal studies. For instance, some cattle develop diabeteslike symptoms when infected with the FOOT AND MOUTH DISEASE virus. Also, investigators have discovered a variant of the encephalo-myocarditis virus (see ENCEPHALOMYOCARDITIS VIRUS INFEC-TION) that produces diabetes in mice. This virus multiplies almost exclusively in the cells of the islets of Langerhans, and as a result of its action the infected mice produce reduced amounts of insulin, develop sugar in the blood and urine, and show marked increases of thirst and appetite. Here, too, there is a genetic factor, the mice of some strains being far more likely than those of others to develop diabetes when infected with the virus. Other investigators have looked for evidence of diabetes in mice infected with certain coxsackie viruses, but although the viruses do attack the pancreas, the appearance of diabeteslike symptoms is not so clear-cut.

EASTERN EQUINE ENCEPHALITIS. See EQUINE EN-CEPHALITIS.

ECHO VIRUS INFECTION. See COXSACKIE OR ECHO VIRUS INFECTION.

EEE. See EQUINE ENCEPHALITIS.

EMC. See ENCEPHALOMYOCARDITIS VIRUS INFECTION.

ENCEPHALITIS. Inflammation of the brain, or encephalitis, is the chief symptom of some virus diseases, a regular feature of others, and an occasional complication of a great many more. The signs of this disorder range from headache and drowsiness, through personality changes (moodiness, excitability), sensory disturbances (such as hallucination), and partial paralysis, to coma, convulsions, and death.

Among the true encephalitises* are several varieties of ARBOVIRUS DISEASE, namely the CALIFORNIA, EQUINE, ST. LOUIS, and TICK-BORNE ENCEPHALITISES. The diseases in which encephalitis is a more or less regular feature are RABIES, YELLOW FEVER, and POLIO. And among the many diseases which it occasionally complicates are MEASLES, MUMPS, and CHICKEN POX.

Also encephalitis is a rare, but most troublesome, aftereffect of SMALLPOX vaccination. REYE'S SYNDROME, a form of encephalitis accompanied by liver malfunction, sometimes follows attacks of virus diseases, most notably chicken pox and INFLUENZA. And, finally, encephalitis often occurs in conjunction with MENINGITIS.

Although most cases of encephalitis are virus-caused, bacteria and other organisms also are capable of bringing it about. The disorder also may be produced by chemical poisons, such as arsenic and mercury, and it may result from malnutrition.

Encephalitis is sometimes popularly characterized as "sleeping sickness," but that term is rarely appropriate for the condition since overexcitability and convulsions are as likely to occur as paralysis and coma. Only one form of encephalitis, known as encephalitis lethargica, might properly be termed a sleeping sickness since it produces a kind of general somnolence and stupor. Although encephalitis lethargica occurred widely in the 1920s—it is thought by some to have been an aftereffect of the influenza epidemic of 1918—it is rarely observed today. (In this discussion we are not, of course, talking about the true African sleeping sickness, which is caused by a protozoan and spread by the tsetse fly.)

Viral encephalitises are generally difficult to treat. Fortunately most mild cases do not require hospitalization, and recovery, though slow, is usually complete. In more severe cases, surgery may be called for to relieve pressure on the brain. Fatalities are not uncommon, and aftereffects such as mental retardation and partial paralysis occur with some frequency.

*The officially sanctioned plural form of the word "encephalitis" is "encephalitides," but this seems so artificial that the more natural "encephalitises" is used throughout this book.

ENCEPHALOMYOCARDITIS (EMC) VIRUS INFECTION. The encephalomyocarditis viruses are a group of viruses* that normally infect small wild animals, but occasionally attack human beings. In mice, monkeys, and squirrels, the animals most frequently infected, these viruses cause infections of the central nervous system and the muscles of the heart (as the name suggests, "encephalo-" meaning brain, "myo-" muscle, and "card-" heart).

In man these viruses are thought to produce ENCEPHALITIS or MENINGITIS, and disorders ranging from a mild feverish illness to a POLIO-like paralytic disease have been tentatively attributed to their action. Several epidemics of human disease are thought to have been due to one or more of these viruses, but the evidence is not conclusive. One such epidemic occurred among American troops in Manila in 1945. Nevertheless, it is generally assumed that these viruses do not represent a major source of human illness.

ENDOCARDITIS. See HEART DISEASE.

EPIDEMIC MYALGIA. See PLEURODYNIA.

EQUINE ENCEPHALITIS (EQUINE ENCEPHALOMYELITIS). There are three well-known mosquito-borne "brain fevers" or encephalitises (see ENCEPHALITIS) that affect both men and horses in annual summertime *epidemics* in North and South America, known as Eastern, Western, and Venezuelan equine encephalitis—or EEE, WEE, and VEE, respectively. They are caused by different viruses and vary in their severity, but all three diseases produce much the same set of symptoms in men and in horses. In man these range from headache, drowsiness, and fever to coma, convulsions, and occasionally death. With the horse the symptoms are more severe ("agonizing") and almost always fatal. Neither man nor horse is the chief host of these viruses, however, for they all mainly infect wild birds and rodents. The viruses are carried among their wild hosts by mosquitoes, and men and horses are infected only when they happen to be bitten by mosquitoes carrying the virus.

For man, Eastern equine encephalitis is the most severe. Death rates as high as 65 percent have been recorded. Infants and children are the hardest hit, with the elderly also quite susceptible.

---

*Included are the viruses designated EMC, ME, Columbia-SK, and Mengo virus.

The symptoms begin suddenly, with headache, fever, and vomiting. Sometimes, then, there is a brief respite, but within a day the attack resumes, now with a fever approaching 106°F and increased signs of central nervous system involvement, ranging from drowsiness to coma, from twitching movements to severe convulsions. Stiffness of the neck and spasticity also are observed. Generally the face becomes puffy, hands and legs swell, and in infants the fontanel bulges. The white cell count is high, and the cerebrospinal fluid, which is under great pressure, contains many white cells.

When death occurs, it often comes within three to five days— sometimes it is a bit later; otherwise symptoms generally last one to three weeks, and then slowly subside. Even children who survive are likely to be permanently impaired; some 60 percent are emotionally disturbed, mentally retarded, paralyzed to some degree, or periodically subject to convulsions.

With increasing age—up to a point—symptoms become less severe and chances for survival increase. But the elderly and feeble, too, are hard hit. Those of middle years generally recover completely, with no aftereffects. Even among children, however, mild cases with complete recovery do occur. And in every epidemic there are many *inapparent infections*, as indicated by the detection of *antibodies* to the virus in apparently healthy individuals.

Western equine encephalitis is somewhat milder, with a mortality rate of 10 to 15 percent. Practically speaking, the disease is almost indistinguishable from the Eastern variety. Fever and drowsiness are almost invariably present; restlessness and irritability are common. But the full range of disturbance, including coma, convulsions, and death, does occur, though less frequently than with EEE. Here recovery tends to come more quickly, usually after five to ten days, and permanent damage is less likely. Only infants under one year are prone to serious, permanent impairment, but older children may experience recurring convulsions for some time.

The Venezuelan disease is the mildest of the group. Most people experience only a feverish illness, without symptoms of encephalitis— although this does occur in enough people to characterize the disease— and death rates are under 1 percent. Often the disease is simply flu-like, with headache, fever, nausea, chills, and muscle and bone aches lasting three or four days. Yet, the full range of encephalitic symptoms may be found in some patients in any epidemic.

Eastern equine encephalitis occurs up and down the Atlantic coast of North and South America, from Argentina to New England. Epidemics occur in late summer, in some areas every year. But on the whole the disease is uncommon.

Not so the Western disease. It was first found in the Central Valley of California and appears to be *endemic* there, with cases occurring nearly every year. But it is found elsewhere—in 1941 an epidemic hit more than 3,000 people in the north central United States and Canada. Epidemics flare up from time to time in virtually every part of the United States and Canada. Every year, in the United States alone, some 20 to 40 cases are confirmed, even in the absence of an epidemic.

Originally confined to Venezuela, which experienced severe epidemics in the early 1960s, VEE has been marching steadily northward, first across Central America, then into Mexico. In 1971 it entered the United States and caused a minor epidemic—about 100 human cases, with one suspected death.

Horses are highly susceptible to all three viruses; death rates of 90 percent in outbreaks are common. Hence these diseases are of great economic importance wherever horses are raised.

The viruses responsible for each of these diseases have been found in a variety of wild birds and small animals; even infected snakes have been observed. Also, mosquitoes of a number of species have been shown to be capable of carrying the viruses from one animal to another. A necessary prerequisite for such transmission is that viruses appear in the blood of the infected animal in sufficient numbers that they can be picked up when the mosquito feeds. This is the case with many of the birds and wild animals infected, although in both horses and man such a condition of *viremia* is not an important part of the disease process. It is for this reason that both horse and human cases are "dead-end" infections—man and horse can become infected, but since they do not undergo viremia, they do not infect others.

It is suspected that under certain circumstances these viruses can be spread in ways other than by mosquito bites. Pheasants confined to single pens rapidly acquire the EEE virus from one another, apparently by ingestion, and it has been reported that the VEE virus can be spread between horses by direct contact. But such cases are thought to be exceptional. There has been no suggestion that any of these diseases can be transmitted from one person to another by direct contact.

Treatment of these encephalitises is generally limited to making the patient as comfortable as possible. Aspirin is used to reduce fever and pain, and other drugs may be employed to halt convulsions in severe cases. Hospitalization is called for if symptoms of encephalitis become acute.

As is true of other mosquito-borne diseases, control of these encephalitises is difficult since the outlawing of DDT and certain other insecticides, and increasing attention is being given to the development of vaccines. Concerns over human health are paramount here, but the damage done to horses is economically significant. *Killed-virus vaccines* that are reasonably effective against all three viruses are available for use in horses, but an early human killed-virus vaccine for VEE proved unacceptable because of severe reactions. An *attenuated-virus vaccine* for VEE was subsequently developed by the United States Army and employed successfully in the epidemic of 1971.

On the basis of symptoms alone, it is impossible to tell these diseases apart—or to tell them from other kinds of encephalitis. Positive identification, then, depends on identification of the causative virus. In fatal cases, tissue samples are taken from the central nervous system on autopsy. Virus isolation here is a definite sign of disease. In live patients, VEE viruses can often be found in blood samples or nose or throat swabs; but with EEE and WEE, viruses in the blood or the upper respiratory tract are much scarcer, and such tests are likely to prove negative. In tests of this kind, the viruses are usually detected by their effect on specific kinds of cells grown in *tissue culture*. Also, it is often possible to measure the rise of antibodies against these viruses in the blood during the course of infection by *serologic tests*.

The viruses are all in the group A arbovirus class (see ARBOVIRUS DISEASE). The virus particles are about 50 nanometers (two millionths of an inch) in diameter and spherical (technically, *icosahedral*) in structure. They contain *RNA*, and are encased in an *outer membrane*.

FIEDLER'S MYOCARDITIS. See COXSACKIE OR ECHO VIRUS INFECTION.

FLU. See INFLUENZA. (But for STOMACH FLU, see GASTRO-ENTERITIS.)

FOOT AND MOUTH DISEASE. Primarily a disease of cattle, foot and mouth disease is occasionally contracted by human beings. In man it produces a rather mild, feverish illness with tiny blisters in the mouth, as well as on and between the fingers and toes.

In animals the disease is much feared because it is so highly contagious and because it affects cattle, our chief source of animal protein. Actually, however, it attacks all cloven-hoofed animals, including pigs, sheep, and goats. The disease takes the form of painful sores in the mouth and on the hoofs, which make it difficult for the animal to feed or move about. Although the disease is rarely fatal, it causes weight loss and decreases in milk production.

Foot and mouth disease does not spread easily to man, and presumably it does so only through cut or abraded skin that comes in direct contact with infected animals. (It has been suggested that the virus can be spread by eating contaminated meat, but this seems unlikely.) In man the disease lasts less than a week, and the sores heal rapidly without leaving scars. The symptoms can resemble those of the so-called hand, foot, and mouth disease, which is caused by a coxsackie virus (see COXSACKIE OR ECHO VIRUS INFECTION). This is not too surprising, since the foot and mouth disease virus is a picornavirus (a small *RNA* virus), as the coxsackie and echo viruses are, and it much resembles them physically.

Veterinary vaccines are available; in man the disease is rare enough and mild enough not to warrant the development of vaccines, or to call for special treatment. Diagnosis is by isolation of the virus from the sores and cultivation of it in tissue cultures. Alternatively, the rise of *antibodies* to the virus can be detected during the course of the disease by *serologic tests*.

FRENCH POLIO. See GUILLAIN-BARRÉ SYNDROME.

GASTROENTERITIS (STOMACH FLU). Gastrointestinal disturbance, ranging from upset stomach to vomiting or diarrhea, is a frequently observed symptom of virus disease. In particular POLIO, and sometimes COXSACKIE OR ECHO VIRUS INFECTION, includes some degree of such disturbance. But there is a brief, common, *epidemic* disease—known colloquially as "stomach flu"—of which this is the chief symptom. In some epidemics the causative agent is identified as a bacterium of some kind; but more often no active agent is found, and the disease is attributed to some unknown virus, simply by default. Recently, however, there is good evidence that several forms of epidemic gastroenteritis are due to infection by particular viral agents.

For example, it now seems that epidemics of gastroenteritis among infants and young children in summer and winter months are due, respectively, to an echo virus and a reovirus-like agent (see REOVIRUS INFECTION). Although the evidence in neither case is conclusive, it does strongly suggest that the virus in question is responsible for many, if not most, of the observed cases of such disease.

Yet, with both these viruses, the number of observed cases of adult gastroenteritis is small, and since many epidemics of gastroenteritis appear to hit all ages equally, it seems likely that some other viral agent, or agents, must be involved. One such agent has been tentatively identified by the use of the electron microscope as a parvovirus, which somewhat resembles the presumed viral agent of infectious HEPATITIS. (Chronic gastroenteritis is generally thought to be a functional disorder and not an infectious disease, but see CROHN'S DISEASE AND ULCERATIVE COLITIS.)

Typically, epidemic gastroenteritis begins abruptly with fever, headache, and malaise; muscle aches may also be observed. But the principal sign, which is usually present almost from the beginning, is stomach distress—vomiting or diarrhea, or both, may be present and, in fact, are likely to be prolonged and debilitating. Yet, serious as the disease is, it is likely to be over as abruptly as it began—after a period of usually under 4 days, thereby giving rise to such popular names for the disease as "24-hour-," "48-hour-," or "3-day virus."

In young, healthy adults the disease not only passes quickly but leaves no lasting effects. In infants, and in the aged and infirm, it is likely to be more insidious, and fatalities, though not common, do occur.

There is no special therapy for gastroenteritis, and until more is known about the causative viruses there can be no vaccines. Nonetheless, since infant diarrhea is a serious disorder, and since there now seem to be some good leads to two of the viruses that cause it, one may hope that development of vaccines in this area will be expedited. It is suspected that transmission of the causative viruses in any case is by the fecal-oral route, so isolation of affected individuals, and extreme care over personal hygiene on the part of those exposed to them, may help in halting local epidemics.

GERMAN MEASLES (RUBELLA). Milder than ordinary MEASLES, and in fact one of the mildest of childhood diseases, German measles would be unremarkable except that it can cause serious birth defects in babies born of mothers who have had the disease during the first few months of pregnancy (*congenital infections*). Fortunately a good vaccine against the disease has been available since 1969. In the United States it is given on a large scale to young children in the hope of eradicating the disease, and its use among young women who have not had the disease is encouraged.

Although German measles is probably many centuries old at least, it was first clearly distinguished from ordinary measles in the 19th century in Germany, where several *epidemics* were carefully investigated (hence the name "German" measles). The connection between the disease and birth defects was not made until 1941. In that year an Australian ophthalmologist, Sir Norman Gregg, noticed an unusually large number of infants with cataracts, heart defects, and other abnormalities. In seeking a possible explanation he recalled an epidemic of German measles the previous year, and careful checking soon revealed that nearly all mothers of the defective children had had the disease during the first three months of pregnancy. This discovery aroused intense interest, not only because it was the first demonstration of a cause of birth defects other than "genetic abnormality," but also because it suggested that at least some birth defects are preventable.

Much investigation in subsequent years has served only to confirm and extend Sir Norman Gregg's observations. It is now well established that German measles during the first trimester of pregnancy can cause the mother to bear a child with any or all of the following defects: brain damage; cardiac malformations; ear abnormalities leading to deafness; cataracts, glaucoma, and other eye disorders; and malfunction of the various internal organs. Life expectancies of many of these infants are below normal, and it is considered likely that many instances of miscarriage and stillbirth are due to extreme abnormality of the fetus caused by this disease. The risk of damage to the fetus is greater the earlier in pregnancy the infection occurs. If rubella is contracted in the first month, nearly half the infants show severe malformations; by the third month the proportion has fallen to 17 percent. The overall statistics show the seriousness of the problem. In the last (1964) major German measles epidemic in the United States, 20,000 children were born with defects traceable to the disease, and another 30,000 were estimated lost as abortions or stillbirths. It is thought that introduction of the vaccine in 1969 headed off a similar epidemic predicted for the early 1970s.

The fact that German measles is caused by a virus was postulated as early as 1914 on the basis of studies with monkeys, but this hypothesis was not confirmed until 1941 when the disease was transmitted to children by means of nasal washings that had been filtered to remove bacteria. In 1962 it was found possible to grow the virus in *tissue culture,* opening the way to preparation of the vaccine.

The first attenuated virus suitable for vaccine use, designated HPV-77, was obtained in 1966, and the first *attenuated-virus vaccine* for the disease was licensed in the United States in 1969. Vaccination does not cause noticeable symptoms in most patients, although some children and slightly more adults experience low fevers, slight rash, and transient joint pains. Viruses can be detected in the throats of vaccinees, but these do not spread even to those with whom the vaccinees come in close contact. Good protection has been shown to be afforded by the vaccine for at least a year; it is thought to last much longer.

There are two schools of thought as to how the vaccine is best used. The first, which has been adopted as official policy in the United States, is that it is best to vaccinate as many children as possible under the age of 12 years. This group has the majority of cases of the disease, and of course the risk of unexpected pregnancies among the vaccinees is minimal. (It is now known that the vaccine viruses can affect a developing fetus in much the same way that ordinary rubella viruses do.) The idea is to hit the disease where it is most common, preventing epidemics and thereby reducing the risk of exposure of unprotected pregnant women. At the same time, all unprotected young women are encouraged to be vaccinated three months before any planned pregnancies. (A simple blood test determines whether or not they have *antibodies* to the virus, resulting from vaccination or earlier infection.) In time, if this policy is followed, the disease should be completely eradicated.

The second approach, which is being tried in Britain and is advocated by some authorities in the United States, is to vaccinate only adolescent girls, including all between 11 and 14. Proponents of this method argue that vaccination of all youngsters is largely wasted effort, since the disease is so mild, whereas concentration on adolescent girls offers them better protection while they are of child-bearing age. They argue further that mass vaccination of the young has failed to eliminate the disease among pregnant women—largely because a few women do acquire the disease from contacts not in the 1-to-12 age group—and that consequently cases of birth defects still occur. With this approach, however, there is increased danger of unexpected pregnancies among the fresh vaccinees, with possibly serious consequences. Furthermore, vaccinating only such a limited group permits the disease to continue unchecked in the population at large and ensures that vaccination of this group will always be necessary.

Thus, although it has been criticized, the accepted policy in the United States—mass vaccination of children and voluntary vaccination of young women—appears on balance to be the wisest course. There is no doubt that it has materially improved the situation. In 1969, the last year before introduction of the vaccine, there were 58,000 cases of rubella reported in the United States (and probably many times that many unreported); in 1974, only 12,000 cases were reported, a decline of almost 80 percent. And better yet, in 1974 only 45 children were born with birth defects due to German measles (compared to the thousands born each year before the vaccine). In all, some 55 million children have received the vaccine—34 states require inoculation before admission to school. Yet, as is also the case with measles and polio, there is some evidence that the pace of vaccination has slowed in the last year or two, and public health officials warn that if the percentage of vaccinated children falls too low, the risk of major epidemics will again be high. Clearly, mass immunization programs must be maintained until the disease has been eradicated.

Typically, the symptoms of rubella appear 16 to 18 days after exposure, though the *incubation period* may run anywhere from 2 to 3 weeks. In youngsters the rash is often the first sign of illness. It consists of pinkish raised spots, lighter than those of ordinary, or "red," measles. These may merge to form large blotches or remain discrete. They form first on the face and move downward rapidly, much more so than those of ordinary measles. Within a day they begin to fade, leaving no mark, with the first often gone before the last appear. Symptoms of a slight cold may also be present during this initial period, which lasts only 2 or 3 days. Almost invariably the rash is accompanied or preceded by a low fever and enlargement of lymph nodes in the neck and behind the ears. These swollen tender glands are a characteristic sign of the disease. In adolescents and young adults the whole process is likely to be more severe— headache, fever, and cold symptoms often appear before the rash, which is itself apt to be extensive, and a transient ARTHRITIS sometimes occurs. ENCEPHALITIS is a rare complication, even rarer than is the case with measles, and there are none of the secondary bacterial infections that so often complicate measles. Even with adults, the illness is mild and over with quickly.

Viruses are found in the nose and throat for a few days before and after the rash, and it seems likely that infection is chiefly by airborne droplets. These may be more abundant when there are coldlike symptoms. Because the clinical course is so much like that of ordinary measles, it is assumed that the two viruses operate in much the same way.

Most cases of German measles are so mild that no treatment at all is necessary, not even bed rest, though the more vigorous activities of the child should probably be curtailed, and he should be confined to the home during the period of rash or other clinical symptoms. Aspirin may be given for headache and fever, and more extensive aspirin therapy is undertaken when signs of arthritis appear. The mild encephalitis that sometimes arises calls for medical attention.

The chief problem, really, is to prevent contact of the infected child with any unprotected women in the first few months of pregnancy, but since the child may be infective before the symptoms appear, this is all but impossible. Therefore, until measles vaccination becomes so widespread that the disease is no longer prevalent, it is up to young women themselves to seek vaccination before pregnancy if they have not had the disease.

Rubella is found everywhere. It is *endemic* in large cities, with outbreaks occurring sporadically rather than cyclically, as is the case with true measles. Where the disease is epidemic, outbreaks occur in a six- to nine-year cycle. The disease tends to strike in the spring, though fall and winter outbreaks are not unknown.

For a childhood disease, rubella usually hits somewhat late—later than regular measles, for example, so that it is often thought to be a second, milder attack of that disease. Except for congenital infections, of course, German measles rarely strikes infants under one year; it peaks among older children, and attacks adolescents and young adults with some frequency. This late attack is probably due to a low infectivity of the virus, which limits its spread and delays the time the average person encounters it.

Congenital rubella, rubella of the fetus, contracted from the mother in utero, is very different from the benign disease of the older child. The effects already described may be severe, resulting in shortened life expectancy and lifelong physical or mental impairment. It is not known precisely how the virus causes the abnormal development of the fetus, but it is quite clear that it crosses the placental barrier and multiplies within the cells of the developing infant. In tissue cultures the virus shows the unusual property of persisting in cells without destroying them, while interfering with normal cell division. It is presumed that something similar happens to the fetus—that cells of organs undergoing development are invaded and fail to divide as expected, thereby disordering the normal process of maturation. In agreement with this hypothesis is the observation that infants with congenital rubella commonly weigh less than normal infants, a possible indication of an overall reduction in number of body cells.

The precise cells invaded by the virus probably determine what defects occur, but there is undoubtedly also a dependence on the phase of development of the fetus; different organs undergo their most rapid development at different times, and their susceptibility to the virus may vary according to their degree of development. In this connection it is observed that different effects follow infection at different stages of gestation: cataracts often occur after an attack in the sixth week; deafness after one in the ninth.

The newborn infant congenitally infected with rubella is likely to be still in a state of active infection, that is, containing viruses in many body organs and emitting viruses in urine and throat and nasal secretions. In some cases even children without observable defects are congenitally infected and shedders of viruses. Peculiarly enough, high levels of viruses persist in the face of equally high levels of antibodies. (It can be assumed that the viruses first invade cells before development of the antibodies and then persist within cell lines where they do not encounter the antibodies.)

Viruses in such cases are likely to remain for some months before they finally disappear. In fact, they may be shed for six months or more, making the affected child a potent source of infection. (It is possible that in the past, before congenital rubella was known, such carrier children played a part in maintaining rubella epidemics.) In certain isolated tissues of the body, viruses may persist for even longer periods. They have been found in cataracts, for example, after three years.

Treatment of children with rubella defects varies greatly, of course, depending on the nature and severity of the damage. The worse difficulties are encountered by newborns with extensive reddish patches caused by bleeding into the skin (a condition known as thrombocytopenic purpura). This symptom is often indicative of generalized internal bleeding, and infants exhibiting it have a mortality rate of about 35 percent in the first year; the comparable rate for all other children with rubella defects is 10 percent. With many congenitally infected infants there is a marked improvement after about six months, when the virus disappears, and the child then often begins to gain weight for the first time at a normal pace. Many infants with minor defects, such as partial deafness, need no special treatment after this period and mature quite normally. Others do equally well after removal of cataracts or surgical correction of heart defects. Some children, however, require special care for many years.

Obviously, the key to control of congenital rubella is prevention. Hence the emphasis on vaccination for women planning pregnancies. Once a pregnancy is under way, the matter is more serious. Vaccination during pregnancy is not advised because of the possible effect of the vaccine viruses on the fetus. In one study of pregnant women inadvertently given the vaccine, viruses and some damage to developing organs were found in a small percentage of the fetuses. *Gamma globulin* is sometimes given to pregnant women in the hope of preventing infection, but there is no clear evidence that it is effective. There is little else that can be done, however, except to try to prevent exposure to known or suspected rubella cases.

If a woman in her early months of pregnancy does contract German measles, the problem is clearly acute. Giving gamma globulin at this point, to prevent damage to the fetus, is probably ineffective, according to most expert opinion. Therapeutic abortion in such cases is clearly called for. Otherwise the risk of bearing an infected child is very high. In one study, 68 percent of fetuses obtained from therapeutic abortion performed on women infected with rubella in the first trimester showed clear signs of infection. When legal, religious, or medical reasons preclude abortion, even in cases where the rubella infection is confirmed, large doses of gamma globulin may be resorted to.

Under many circumstances, exact diagnosis of German measles is not important; the disease in children is simply too mild to worry about. Thus, diagnosis is often accomplished simply by reviewing the symptoms. It is difficult only to differentiate the disease from mild cases of ordinary measles (in which the Koplik's spots may be absent) and from infectious MONONUCLEOSIS and COXSACKIE OR ECHO VIRUS INFECTION, which are sometimes accompanied by rash. With pregnant women, however, as well as the children they may have been exposed to, the matter is more serious. In such instances, as with newborns suspected of being congenitally infected, accurate diagnosis is all important. And such accurate diagnosis can be obtained only by laboratory procedures.

The best laboratory test for rubella virus is actual isolation of the virus from the throat (or other areas) and cultivation of it in tissue cultures of various kinds. In some types of cells used in such cultures the virus causes characteristic damage, which permits positive identification; in other cells the virus causes no visible effect, but it does interfere with the growth of other viruses that would produce such effects, and in this case the lack of visible cell damage indicates that the rubella virus is present.

Rubella can also be diagnosed in the laboratory by detection of a marked rise in levels of antibodies to the virus in the blood as the disease proceeds. For such *serologic tests,* blood samples are drawn when the patient first becomes ill, and again in two to four weeks.

The laboratory animal most susceptible to the virus is the monkey—though other animals can be infected under rather special circumstances—and monkey cells were first used to cultivate the virus. Viruses for vaccine use are now grown in cultures of cells from various organs of several kinds of animals.

The rubella virus itself has not been studied much until recently. Apparently it is a fairly large *RNA* virus, variously reported as anywhere from 50 to 130 nanometers in diameter, with 70 nanometers (three millionths of an inch) probably a good figure. The somewhat irregular particles are surrounded by an *outer membrane* and said to resemble the myxoviruses, among which this virus is sometimes classed. Only one form of the virus is known.

GLANDULAR FEVER. See MONONUCLEOSIS.

GOUT. See CONNECTIVE TISSUE DISEASE.

GREEN MONKEY DISEASE. See MARBURG DISEASE.

GUILLAIN-BARRÉ SYNDROME (ACUTE IDIOPATHIC POLY-NEURITIS, ASCENDING PARALYSIS, FRENCH POLIO). A neurological disorder characterized by a temporary paralysis that moves upward through the body, Guillain-Barré syndrome is a disease of unknown cause. It occurs occasionally following infections, vaccinations, and surgery. Recovery is usually complete, and the death rate is low—5 percent. Symptoms begin with weakness and loss of sensation in the feet and legs. A paralysis then begins and gradually extends upward. When the breathing muscles are attacked, an artificial respirator may be needed—this is the chief life-threatening action of the disorder. In time the speech may be affected. After a week to ten days the symptoms begin to recede. A very few victims are left permanently paralyzed.

Guillain-Barré syndrome—it is named for two French physicians who first described it in 1916—has been observed after a number of different infections, chiefly viral. In at least one instance, it has followed a CYTOMEGALOVIRUS INFECTION. A number of cases arose in the wake of the swine-flu vaccination campaign of 1977, and were instrumental in bringing the campaign to an end (see INFLUENZA).

HAND, FOOT, AND MOUTH DISEASE. See COXSACKIE OR ECHO VIRUS INFECTION.

HEART DISEASE. Cardiovascular disease, malfunction of the heart and blood vessels, is the leading cause of death in the United States and other highly developed countries. In the United States more than half of all deaths fall into this category, most of them due to heart attack or stroke. The underlying conditions responsible for most cardiovascular disease are high blood pressure, hypertension, and hardening of the arteries, arteriosclerosis. What is responsible for hypertension and arteriosclerosis, however, is still somewhat uncertain. Diet, heredity, and life style have all been implicated, but areas of mystery remain. A few authorities suspect that viruses are involved, but this is generally considered unlikely. There are, on the other hand, several uncommon but serious heart ailments in which viruses are known to be involved, chiefly inflammations of the muscles, membranes, and valves of the heart.

The chief cardiovascular defect—the one responsible for most cases of heart attack and stroke—is the clogging of the arteries with fatty deposits, a process known as atherosclerosis.* A rare complication of atherosclerosis is inflammation of the affected artery, which much resembles the arterial inflammation observed with some forms of CONNECTIVE TISSUE DISEASE. Since connective tissue disease is often thought to be due to a kind of SLOW VIRUS DISEASE, by extension atherosclerosis sometimes too is placed in this category. The idea is that a virus which might be extremely difficult to detect would chronically infect the connective tissue of the arterial wall and initiate the changes that would result in atherosclerosis. But there is no evidence that any such infection occurs.

Where viruses are known to be involved is in acute invasions of the heart and its surrounding membrane. Whereas such invasions are most uncommon, at least compared to the many cases of chronic heart disease, they do occur and can be life-threatening. The various conditions reported are as follows: myocarditis, inflammation of the heart muscle, which can be a serious matter in adults and is often fatal in infants; endocarditis, inflammation of the heart valves, which generally is of bacterial origin, but which can be viral; and pericarditis, inflammation of the heart membrane, which can be painful, but which is less likely to have serious consequences than either of the other two. The viruses responsible for INFLUENZA, MUMPS, POLIO, and MONONUCLEOSIS have all been responsible for causing one or more of these conditions, but it is the coxsackie viruses (see COXSACKIE OR ECHO VIRUS INFECTION) that are the most frequent offenders. An *epidemic*, often fatal myocarditis of infants has frequently been traced to coxsackie virus infections.

Diagnosis of acute viral heart disease is complicated by the difficulty of detecting viruses within the heart, although the presence of viruses elsewhere, such as in the stool, may indicate an active viral infection, as does a sharp rise of *antibodies* in the blood, which can be revealed by

---

*Needless to say, the resemblance between the terms "arteriosclerosis" and "atherosclerosis" causes considerable confusion, but the terms can hardly be avoided.

serologic tests. In fatal cases, samples of heart tissue can be taken at autopsy, and viruses can then be cultivated from them in various ways, confirming the diagnosis.

In acute virus infection of the heart little can be done to combat the virus directly. But the physician can use (1) cortisone and related steroids to reduce inflammation, and (2) digitalis and other heart drugs to control the action of the heart and minimize the risk of heart failure.

HEMORRHAGIC FEVER. "Hemorrhagic fever" is a general term referring to any acute feverish disease accompanied by rash, oozing of blood from the gums and other mucous membranes, and, frequently, bleeding of the internal organs. Many virus diseases, such as MEASLES, show the blotchy rashes characteristic of more severe hemorrhagic disease, but the phrase "hemorrhagic fever" is usually reserved for certain rather severe diseases of which hemorrhagic signs and fever are the chief symptoms. They chiefly affect wild rodents and only occasionally man. YELLOW FEVER and DENGUE are similar to these diseases in some respects, but are different enough to be recognized as separate diseases.

There is a whole group of hemorrhagic fevers. All show much the same pattern of symptoms, but each is localized in a particular geographical area of its own. Some are known to be caused by different, but related, viruses; with others, the causative virus has not yet been isolated.

Perhaps the most thoroughly studied of these as a disease, and certainly one of the most serious, is "Russian hemorrhagic fever with renal (kidney) syndrome," known also as "hemorrhagic nephrotic nephritis" ("nephr-" also refers to kidney). This disease has been known since the 1930s. It is widely spread across eastern Europe and Russia, taking a severe form in the Soviet Far East, and a milder one in European Russia and adjoining countries. Besides the usual hemorrhagic signs of rash, bleeding from the gums, and lowered white-cell count, this disease is characterized by heavy damage to the kidneys. This makes itself felt in intense pain in the kidney area and a diminution, frequently a complete drying up, of the urine. What urine appears is likely to be cloudy with protein and damaged cells; it may contain blood. In areas where the disease is severe, the death rate approaches 15 percent.

It seems quite clear that this disease is carried by a virus, though the virus has not been isolated. It also seems clear that the human victims of the disease catch the virus in some way from small, wild rodents, which inhabit the areas where it is found—voles are probably the responsible rodents in much of Russia. And although it is possible that the virus is carried from rodent to man by the bite of a tick or mite, it has been very difficult to prove this. It is now suspected by Russian authorities that the virus is spread via rodent urine or feces, which the person contacts either directly or as dried dusts admitted to the air.

Although this disease occurs at various times of the year, it is most prevalent in summer and autumn. Also, it is mainly rural—typical victims are farmers, foresters, and fieldworkers of various kinds.

Besides this hemorrhagic fever with renal syndrome, three other, more typical hemorrhagic fevers are known in Russia. These are Omsk, Crimean, and Central Asian hemorrhagic fevers. None of them causes kidney disturbance, and in their symptoms of rash and intestinal and external bleeding, they are quite similar. Central Asian hemorrhagic fever is the most severe; it is characterized by massive bleeding and severe damage to the gastrointestinal tract—vomiting of blood is common. Both the Omsk and the Crimean varieties of the disease display milder signs. Omsk fever is likely to be accompanied by respiratory distress, usually bronchitis, sometimes pneumonia; Crimean fever, by nervous system involvement, headache, drowsiness, sometimes delirium and hallucinations.

Central Asian hemorrhagic fever is not a serious health problem at present, though it was so in the past. Crimean fever is now endemic in various areas along the Black Sea, including parts of Russia, Romania, and Bulgaria, but it apparently no longer occurs in the Crimea. Omsk fever is still found in the Omsk area of Siberia. It is the only one of the Russian hemorrhagic fevers of which the causative virus has actually been isolated and studied. The virus is closely related to that which causes Russian spring-summer encephalitis (see TICK-BORNE ENCEPHALITIS).

The Omsk virus, two types of which are known, has been isolated from rodents and ticks, as well as from human patients, and there is no doubt that the virus is conveyed to its human victims by tick bites—the disease is not contagious by other routes. The chief victims are agricultural workers and handlers of muskrats and muskrat pelts. The Central Asian and Crimean hemorrhagic fevers too are carried by ticks, but the former is—uniquely among this group of viruses—also spread by direct contact among human beings, possibly via discharged blood heavily laden with viruses.

Closely related to the Russian hemorrhagic fevers is the Kyasanur Forest disease of India. This disease was first observed in 1957, though it was later discovered that cases had occurred two years earlier. The disease is *epidemic* among monkeys in the Kyasanur Forest in the Indian state of Mysore. This disease, too, is transferred to man by ticks; and the virus, which has been isolated, is closely related to the Omsk hemorrhagic fever virus. The illness is a feverish one, accompanied initially by back pain, headache, and nausea. Soon bleeding begins from the nose and gums. Although in some epidemics a rash has appeared in the back of the mouth, the skin remains clear. Death rates of about 5 percent are observed.

A Korean hemorrhagic fever also is known, one which caused considerable disease among American troops during the Korean War. Recent work suggests that the virus is one which normally infects a mouse, and that it is transmitted not by a tick, but by contact with mouse excreta, as is the virus of Russian hemorrhagic fever with renal syndrome.

Bolivian and Argentinian hemorrhagic fevers are caused by two related viruses called Machupo virus and Junin virus after the river and town, respectively, near which each was first found. Both infect rodents, and the Junin virus is thought to be carried to man by a mite, but no *vector* has been found for the Machupo virus, and it is thought that this virus too is spread by rodent excreta. So-called hemorrhagic fevers of Thailand, South Vietnam, and the Philippines are due to the dengue and chikungunya viruses (see DENGUE).

There are no cures for any of the hemorrhagic fevers. Bed rest is almost always required, and the more severe diseases warrant hospitalization. Blood loss from hemorrhaging is obviously a serious problem, and it must be dealt with by a physician. Frequent blood transfusions may be necessary.

Nor are there vaccines for these diseases. Hence, control must be accomplished by way of the rodents that harbor the virus or the ticks that carry them to man. Clearing rodents away from the vicinity of human dwellings can be an important step, as is warning fieldworkers and woodsmen not to sleep on the ground. Insecticides can obviously play a role where ticks are involved.

In those cases in which the viruses have been isolated, classification is possible. Because the Omsk hemorrhagic fever and Kyasanur Forest disease viruses are related to the Russian spring-summer encephalitis virus, a known arbovirus (see ARBOVIRUS DISEASE), these seem to be safely in that category. The Machupo and Junin viruses, however, are related to the Tacaribe virus, which infects bats and mosquitoes in Trinidad, and though these three viruses were once also categorized as arboviruses, they are now tentatively placed in a new group, the arenaviruses, along with the LYMPHOCYTIC CHORIOMENINGITIS and LASSA FEVER viruses. These viruses have the properties of infecting rodents for long periods and of spreading to man without the aid of an insect or other arthropod vector. On the basis of their mode of spread to humans, it might seem that the viruses of Korean hemorrhagic fever and Russian hemorrhagic fever with renal syndrome belong to the same group, but until the viruses are actually found this cannot be determined.

HEMORRHAGIC NEPHROTIC NEPHRITIS. See HEMORRHAGIC FEVER.

HEPATITIS (JAUNDICE). Hepatitis, or inflammation of the liver, is signaled by stomach upset and diarrhea, tenderness or pain in the upper abdomen, and jaundice*—a yellowing of the skin and the whites of the eyes. Some viruses, most conspicuously that of YELLOW FEVER, cause hepatitis along with their other symptoms, but there are two virus diseases—the symptoms of which are virtually indistinguishable—in which hepatitis is the major effect, and it is these two diseases that are usually referred to as "hepatitis." (Although hepatitis is generally the result of virus infection, it may also be caused by other infectious agents; by certain drugs, such as chlorpromazine; and by the action of toxic chemicals, like chloroform and carbon tetrachloride.)

The so-called infectious hepatitis, now known increasingly as hepatitis A, is spread through personal contact, consumption of raw seafood, or drinking contaminated water. *Serum* hepatitis, or hepatitis B, is transmitted chiefly by blood transfusions and the use of contaminated hypodermic needles. Because some virus-caused hepatitis cannot be attributed to either of the known hepatitis viruses—or any other identifiable viruses, for that matter—some authorities postulate the existence of a still unisolated hepatitis C virus.

Even though hepatitis A is itself not uncommon, it is hepatitis B that represents a major medical problem. As many as a million carriers of the virus are thought to exist in the United States alone—100 million worldwide—and for a time the threat of serum hepatitis seriously challenged the entire blood donor program. Fortunately, new techniques (based on research that was honored by a Nobel Prize in 1976) permit the screening of blood and the identification of contaminated supplies. Also, there is hope that a new kind of vaccine may be effective against the virus,

---

*Although the words "hepatitis" and "jaundice" are sometimes used synonymously, it is preferable to restrict "jaundice" to the skin discoloration (the word comes from the same root as the French "jaune," meaning yellow) and to use "hepatitis" for the underlying condition. Jaundice, which is often a sign of hepatitis, can result from other causes, such as blockage of the bile duct; and, conversely, though hepatitis is usually accompanied by jaundice, the disorder can occur without noticeable skin discoloration.

and a new treatment shows promise in early tests. These developments are especially important because the hepatitis B virus is thought to be involved also in the initiation of liver CANCER.

In spite of the similarities of the two forms of hepatitis, the respective *incubation periods* are quite different. With hepatitis A the symptoms begin some two to six weeks after exposure; with the B variety they take two to six months. In either case, the first signs are likely to be a malaise, or lassitude, and a loss of appetite. At this time the patient may develop a marked distaste for fatty foods and, if he smokes, an aversion to tobacco. Soon come rather more severe symptoms, such as headache, nausea, vomiting, a light fever, and possibly diarrhea. After these early signs have persisted for a week or two, and the patient may have begun to feel somewhat better, the jaundice begins.

Usually the yellow coloration appears first in the eyes; then it becomes noticeable in the face, the trunk, and the limbs, in that order. The urine too may become dark. Generally the jaundice is accompanied by a resurgence of fever and gastrointestinal disturbance (see GASTRO-ENTERITIS), and by this time the liver is usually tender and sore to the touch. Often this period is characterized by the patient's feeling great fatigue.

The observed jaundice is caused by the appearance in the blood of the pigment bilirubin, which is produced by the liver from waste hemoglobin and normally sent into the intestines as part of the bile. As a result of this shifting of the flow of billirubin, the stools generally become light-colored when jaundice appears. Even in the absence of noticeable jaundice, sensitive tests can detect increased levels of bilirubin in the blood, and other tests may reveal liver malfunction during this phase of the illness.

Typically the period of jaundice lasts for a month or more, with gradually moderating symptoms. Heavy and prolonged jaundice is usually a bad sign, as it may signal permanent liver damage. Except when liver damage does result, recovery is complete, though temporary relapses may occur. Fatalities are not unknown—death rates among young adults are one or two per thousand cases, and they are higher among the elderly and those with liver damage from other causes, such as alcoholism. In children the disease is milder, often much milder, and a great many childhood infections go completely unrecognized.

Although the overall course of the illness is virtually identical in both forms of hepatitis, the rate at which the process unfolds is often slower in hepatitis B. Also, that disorder is less likely to be accompanied by heavy fever, but it may produce ARTHRITIS-like symptoms among its effects.

It is often possible to diagnose hepatitis on the basis of the symptoms alone—the combination of jaundice, mild fever, gastrointestinal disturbance, and tenderness in the area of the liver is usually unmistakable. But when jaundice does not appear the matter may be more difficult. A number of blood tests and other clinical tests* are useful in detecting liver disease whether or not jaundice is present. Now, also, with increased knowledge about the viruses that cause hepatitis, newer diagnostic procedures are becoming available.

The conventional treatment for hepatitis is bed rest, generally maintained until blood bilirubin levels fall to normal. Hospitalization is required only in extreme cases. To minimize demands on the liver, some physicians recommend special diets, which typically proscribe fried and greasy foods and alcoholic beverages. Steroid therapy has been employed in severe cases, but is not used routinely. Still under development are several experimental procedures, discussed below, which are based on studies of the respective viruses.

The hepatitis A virus, the agent of infectious hepatitis, is chiefly spread by direct contact between individuals or through contamination with fecal matter. It has been amply shown that the virus is released in the stools and then, by one of these mechanisms, infects succeeding victims orally. The disease spreads quickly within households and among people who come in close contact with one another. The virus also passes from person to person in food and water. Kitchen workers have been implicated in many hepatitis epidemics, and outbreaks have been traced to contaminated water supplies. It is also documented that a number of people have been infected by eating raw shellfish (mainly oysters and clams) caught in areas that have been contaminated by sewage runoff.

Presumably the virus passes down the digestive tract, multiplies in the intestines, like the POLIO virus and the echo and coxsackie virus (see COXSACKIE OR ECHO VIRUS INFECTION), and then finds its way to the liver via the bloodstream. The stage of prejaundice illness doubtless represents the effects of *viremia* and intestinal multiplication, whereas jaundice, liver sensitivity, and other late signs are marks of liver

---

*Among the most used tests are those for certain enzymes—namely, serum alkaline phosphatase and serum glutamic oxalacetic and pyruvic transaminases—which become positive with liver damage. Also, thymol turbidity and cephalin floculation tests are run to judge liver function, and levels of bilirubin in blood and urine are measured to follow the course of the disease.

attack. In some people, however, the virus enters the body, multiplies in the intestines, and then passes out in the stools without ever managing to reach the liver and cause true hepatitis. Such infections, of course, are *inapparent*.

In 1973 what is presumed to be the causative virus of hepatitis A was found by microscopic examination of stools. Using *antibodies*, which caused the virus particles to clump together and be more easily visible, investigators found numerous small particles, 27 nanometers in diameter (about one millionth of an inch). These particles much resemble those of the parvoviruses, a family of small *DNA*-containing viruses that previously had been implicated only in animal illnesses.

So far researchers have failed to grow the hepatitis A virus in hens' eggs or *tissue culture,* a step that must precede the making of a vaccine. But recently the virus has been found to infect marmosets, a kind of South American monkey, and this is the first known animal host other than man. Using both viruses and antibodies obtained from marmosets, laboratory workers can now use *serologic tests* to confirm the presence of hepatitis A viruses and antibodies in patients, a development that makes possible much firmer diagnoses.

In spite of the absence of a vaccine, the effectiveness of *gamma globulin* as a preventive measure seems well documented. It is given as soon as exposure to the virus is established. Also, several experimental drugs, namely isoprinosine and ribavirin, have shown promise against the virus in certain tests, but these drugs are not in general use. (In fact, recent research has shown that ribavirin can cause congenital abnormalities in hamsters, a finding that raises serious questions about the advisability of using it to treat human disease.)

The hepatitis B virus, which causes serum hepatitis, in most cases does not pass through the alimentary canal at all; rather, it goes—as directly as possible—from the bloodstream of one individual to that of another, where it multiplies and then zeroes in on the liver and produces the hepatitis we observe. A highly unusual property of the virus is that it can remain in the blood for long periods without necessarily attacking the liver. This property accounts for the long incubation period of this form of the disease and also explains the large numbers of people who carry the virus without developing signs of illness.

Serum hepatitis was first uncovered during World War II, when it was found that many servicemen given yellow fever vaccine came down with liver disease. Careful investigative work traced this hepatitis to blood serum that had been added to the vaccine during manufacture. It was then realized that earlier outbreaks of hepatitis could be traced to the giving of whole blood or blood products by injection.

In recent years, as blood transfusions have become an increasingly important part of medical and surgical practice, the incidence of serum hepatitis has soared, until it is now recognized as a serious hazard. In the United States some 30,000 people every year develop serum hepatitis from transfusions—posttransfusion hepatitis, as it is sometimes called—besides the vast numbers who carry the virus without developing disease. Of the active cases, it is estimated that some 10 percent end fatally. This matter obviously poses a terrible problem for physicians recommending blood for medical use—without it the patient may be in serious danger; with it, he may contract hepatitis. And the problem has recently been compounded by mounting evidence that the hepatitis B virus may be a causative factor in liver cancer.

One partial solution to the problem has been to limit the blood used to that supplied by volunteers rather than accepting it from paid donors, many of whom have proved to be chronic carriers of the virus. In areas where this practice has been introduced, the incidence of posttransfusion hepatitis has fallen by 50 percent. And new screening procedures, which detect contaminated blood, are presumably having an even greater effect. There is also evidence that improved techniques in handling collected blood (freezing is one) also lower the risk of hepatitis.

Although blood and blood products, such as serum, represent the major way by which hepatitis B is transmitted, other paths do exist. In fact, whenever people routinely puncture the skin with instruments used on more than one person, the disease makes its appearance. Frequent sources of infection are the instruments used by drug addicts, tattoo artists, and ear piercers. The hepatitis B virus seems to be extraordinarily sturdy, and ordinary cold sterilization methods do not inactivate it. What is needed is heating in boiling water for 20 minutes or autoclaving at even higher temperatures.

It seems safe to assume that the hepatitis B virus existed before man took to infecting himself with it by injection; hence there must be other ways by which the virus is spread in nature. One suggestion is that the virus might have been spread by insects, as the arboviruses are (see ARBOVIRUS DISEASE), with the insect in effect acting as a little hypodermic needle and injecting its virus-laden saliva into the blood. There is indeed some evidence now that insects can harbor the virus, but whether or not they can transmit it to human beings has not been determined.

Another possibility is that the virus might be transmitted by the fecal-oral route as the hepatitis A virus is. Although it was at first assumed that hepatitis B did not include a phase of intestinal infection, it now seems likely that some degree of such infection can occur, and evidence of virus spread by direct contact and fecal contamination is growing. Also, there is mounting evidence of hepatitis B virus contamination of shellfish, as occurs with the A virus. Thus it is becoming increasingly clear that, though the virus of hepatitis B is spread chiefly by man himself with his hypodermic needles, the virus can make its own way from man to man.

The discovery that made possible much of the recent progress in hepatitis B research and which won the Nobel Prize for Baruch S. Blumberg of the Institute for Cancer Research, Philadelphia, was the observation he made in 1967 that the blood of hepatitis B patients almost always carries a particular protein *antigen*. This substance, which Blumberg dubbed the Australia antigen* because he had first detected it four years before in the blood of an Australian aborigine, has now been shown to be composed of the chief building block of the surface layer of the hepatitis B virus particles. When alone, the antigen forms spheres 20 nanometers in diameter (one millionth of an inch), as well as long filaments, and it is these two materials that are found in the blood of hepatitis patients.

The significant features of the Australia antigen are that it is relatively easy to detect and that its presence is a fairly good sign that the hepatitis B virus is also present. Thus the antigen facilitates diagnosis of hepatitis, aids in the detection of carriers, and permits the identification of contaminated blood. It is serologic tests based on this antigen that have made possible the screening of all blood intended for human use and the consequent dramatic lowering of incidence of posttransfusion hepatitis. In addition, some still experimental work has been done on the use of antibodies to the Australia antigen as a trap for hepatitis B virus particles—with the aim of removing them from contaminated blood.

But the most attractive prospect concerning Australia antigen is its potential employment as a new kind of vaccine. The expectation is that injecting patients with purified Australia antigen, isolated from the blood of hepatitis patients or carriers, would cause the formation of protective antibodies against both the antigen and the virus itself, thereby conferring protection without causing infection, just as a *killed-virus vaccine* does. Because this is a new departure in vaccine preparation, vaccine makers are moving extremely carefully. First they must be sure that the vaccine

*This material is also known as the hepatitis associated antigen (HAA), and it is now formally designated HBsAg.

does not contain any of the hepatitis B viruses—or even their *nucleic acid*—or the vaccine itself would be infectious. Second, they must verify that there is no other material included in the vaccine that would cause allergic reactions in recipients, the most likely side effect of any vaccine.

Such a roundabout method of vaccine production is called for in this case because the hepatitis B virus has not so far been successfully cultivated in ways that would make mass production of vaccine possible. The need for a vaccine against this virus is doubly great because it has been found that gamma globulin does not exert a protective effect against it as it does against the A virus—although recently a hepatitis B *immune globulin* has become commercially available. Furthermore, the drugs that look promising against the A virus are not active against the B. There is, however, some recent research with *interferon* which suggests that this naturally protective substance will be helpful in eliminating the B virus from chronic carriers.

One interesting sidelight of the discovery of the Australia antigen is that it reinforces the idea of a natural mode of spread of the virus—other than by injection. For not only was the antigen detected in the original Australian aborigine, but it has also subsequently been widely observed in other Asiatics, suggesting a large naturally infected population in the Orient.

What is thought to be the true hepatitis B virus is another substance found in the blood of hepatitis B patients, the so-called Dane particle. Named for its discoverer, D. M. S. Dane of the Bland-Sutton Institute, London, this particle has a diameter of 42 nanometers (some two millionths of an inch), resembles a virus under the electron microscope, and has been shown to carry an enzyme, DNA polymerase, as well as a strand of DNA in its core, all rather clear indications of its virus nature. Thus the two viruses that cause hepatitis are rather different: certainly in size—the B virus is half again as large as the A virus; but also in chemical makeup, as shown by antibody studies. The situation here is therefore not at all like that of polio or INFLUENZA, where the several causative viruses are all closely related. Undoubtedly this difference in the viruses is why the two forms of hepatitis have such different modes of transmission and such different incubation periods (even though the symptoms are much alike).

HERPANGINA. An acute childhood disease, usually of short duration and with no aftereffects, herpangina is characterized by fever, headache, vomiting, sore throat, and a scattering of small sores in the mouth. The disease is contagious and *epidemic,* and confined to the summer months.

It is caused by various coxsackie viruses (see COXSACKIE OR ECHO VIRUS INFECTION).

Herpangina was first recognized as a specific disease in 1920 when an outbreak occurred in St. Louis, but undoubtedly it is much older. The disease is observed with some frequency in many parts of the world.

The first symptoms come on abruptly, after an *incubation period* of four to seven days, with high fever (often 104°F), headache, and vomiting. Stiff neck and pain in the back are noticed by some patients. Abdominal pain is common. Most patients complain of sore throat, and the few scattered sores in the mouth form rapidly; they first appear as pimples, quickly become blisterlike, and then turn to "punched-out" open sores or ulcers. Generally, the open sores are round and grayish and are surrounded by a red halo. The name, incidentally, is a combination of "herpes" and "angina," suggesting blisterlike sores and sharp pain or distress.

Typically, people with the disease are not terribly sick, and all the symptoms disappear in four or five days. Complications are most unusual (infection of the salivary glands, as in MUMPS, has been observed), and patients invariably recover completely.

Most victims of herpangina are under 10 years of age (the one-to-seven age group is hardest hit), but older children and adults are sometimes affected. The disease is spread by mouth-to-mouth contact, by joint use of eating utensils, and by fecal contamination of the surroundings. (Like the other coxsackie viruses, those that cause herpangina multiply in the throat as well as the intestinal tract and are released to some extent in throat secretions, but more abundantly in the stools.)

There is no real treatment for herpangina; the patient is simply made as comfortable as possible and advised to rest. Diagnosis is often made on the basis of the overall symptoms, with the mouth sores a clear sign of the disease.

Herpangina is most easily confused with HERPES, though the sores in the latter disease tend to appear on the lips, gums, and cheeks, whereas in herpangina they are farther back in the mouth or throat. Also, in herpes the sores are likely to be larger and to run together; often the lips or gums are swollen and painful.

Laboratory tests are used to confirm the diagnosis when there is any doubt. Material from stools or throat swabs is inoculated into newborn mice, which develop a characteristic disorder pointing to the presence of coxsackie viruses of the so-called A group—those chiefly associated with herpangina. Often the specific A viruses involved are not further identified, their behavior being much the same in any case, and the large number making identification difficult. Those implicated most frequently in herpangina are A viruses 1 through 6, 8, 10, and 22. Because so many different viruses are involved, the possibility of developing vaccines to prevent herpangina is not good.

HERPES (HERPES SIMPLEX). The recurring cold sore, or fever blister, on the lip is the most familiar manifestation of herpes, but outbreaks also occur on the nose, in the eye, and on the genitals. In most cases such recurrent infections have been preceded by an initial, heavier attack in the same area, accompanied by general illness. Complications of herpes are ENCEPHALITIS, MENINGITIS, and corneal scarring that can produce blindness. Children born of mothers with active genital herpes sometimes experience serious, even fatal, *congenital infections*. There is considerable evidence that genital herpes is a precursor of cervical CANCER. The virus exists in two closely related forms: herpes-1 virus, which causes infection chiefly above the waist, and herpes-2, chiefly below. Several experimental drugs have shown promising activity against both forms of the virus, and work is under way on vaccines.

The word "herpes" is derived from a Greek word meaning "to creep." It was originally applied by the ancient Greeks to what we now call herpes as well as to SHINGLES. (It is really more appropriate to shingles, in which the blisterlike sores move along in successive waves.) In time the two came to be differentiated, with shingles known as "herpes zoster," and herpes of the lip as simple herpes, or "herpes simplex." Although these terms are still employed, there is an increasing tendency to use simply "zoster" and "herpes" for the two diseases.

Nearly everyone is familiar with cold sores—a great many people have them themselves, more or less regularly, and those who do not, have almost surely seen them on others. They form most commonly on the lip, typically at the line where the mucous membrane joins the skin of the face, but they also occur within the mouth, on the nostrils, and even on the ear. Generally the sore is preceded by an itching, burning, or painful sensation in the affected area. Soon the spot turns red and the small blisters form. After a day or two these break, release whatever matter they contain, and then scab over. Within a week the scab falls off, leaving no scar. Repeated outbreaks occur at or very near the same spot, time after time.

Various things seem to trigger the attacks, though they often occur for no discernible reason. Common stimuli are the onset of colds and fevers (leading, of course, to the common names, cold sore and fever blister); others are overexposure to sunlight, emotional upset, tension, hormonal changes such as those of menstruation, consumption of certain foods or drinks, and dosage with particular drugs.

Although the recurrent cold sores of herpes are severely limited in extent, the initial infection is likely to have been widespread, involving much of the mouth area—or the nose or the ear, in rare cases—and to be accompanied by general illness, with fever and much discomfort. There is usually a swelling of nearby lymph glands. The mouth inflammation, or stomatitis, which is the typical circumstance, occurs most commonly in children between the ages of one and three years, though it does happen in older children and adults. Often fever and malaise come first, followed by a soreness and redness of the lips, tongue, and gums. Even the tonsils may be affected. Soon the cold sore blisters appear over most of the irritated area; they quickly become grayish-yellow plaques, which finally turn into ulcers. Pain is likely to subside first, then the sores clear up, and at last the swelling goes down. The whole process may take up to two weeks.

Sometimes milder initial attacks occur, and some people experience cold sores with no recollection of ever having suffered from stomatitis or other more pronounced infection. In fact, some persons who carry *antibodies* to the virus, a good sign of exposure, never experience any symptoms at all.

An occasional complication of primary, or even recurrent, herpes in the facial area is an encephalitis or meningitis. Such brain disturbance can lead in extreme cases to coma, convulsions, and death. At times these brain disorders are caused by herpes infections even when there is no other sign of the infection. Several cases of Bell's palsy, a kind of facial paralysis, have been traced to herpes infections.

Herpes of the eye is much rarer than herpes of the lip, but it is potentially more serious because it can lead to blindness. The initial infection in this case is likely to take the form of an inflammation of the entire conjunctival membrane surrounding the eyeball—a condition known as conjunctivitis—with cold sore blisters on the eyelids and the whole area red and swollen. (Stomatitis may occur at the same time.) The attack generally clears up within a few days—if it has not extended itself to the cornea, the transparent outer covering of the eyeball. When this so-called keratitis, or inflammation of the cornea, occurs, large branching ulcers form and may penetrate deep into the cornea. This process may last for two or three weeks, and the ulcers may persist even longer. These may clear up without permanent scarring, but this is not always the case—the vision may be partially or completely obstructed. Whatever the nature of the initial attack, repeating outbreaks are likely to occur, and they may spread to the cornea whether or not the initial attack has done so. In no case, however, does the general inflammation of the eye area return.

On very rare occasions cold-sore herpes occurs at highly unusual sites in the body, such as the elbow, where the virus happens to be present and enters the skin through small breaks or abrasions. In the primary infections of such "traumatic herpes," the whole localized area becomes inflamed, the usual herpes sores appear, and the patient is ill and feverish for up to a week. In doctors and nurses, traumatic herpes often appears on the finger as a "herpetic whitlow." This is a single, large sore that is very painful and extends deep into the skin, but it is not accompanied by other signs of illness. Such sores are often contaminated by bacteria, chiefly staphylococci.

Another, a very serious form of herpes, occurs when people with eczema encounter the virus. The primary illness then can spread over much of the skin, taking the form of large open sores. The condition, known as eczema herpeticum, can become so extensive that it is fatal. In most cases, however, the patient begins to improve in a week or ten days. Recurrent attacks occur, but they are likely to be less severe.

Although genital herpes is caused by a variant—the so-called herpes-2 virus—of the virus that produces the above disorders, the disease itself is much the same. In both men and women initial and recurring attacks, much like those described, occur on or in the neighborhood of the genital organs. The initial attack begins with swelling, reddening, and pain in the area surrounding the site of infection—at times the inflammation extends over the whole groin, thighs, and buttocks. This is accompanied by a low-grade fever, mild flu-like symptoms, and swelling of the lymph glands in the groin. The small, blisterlike sores soon appear over much of the inflamed area, and as in primary herpes stomatitis, they rapidly become grayish yellow and ulcerous. The typical infection lasts two weeks. In this area too, mild, even *inapparent infections* can occur. In recurrent attacks only the small blisters appear, in a very limited area; they quickly scab over and heal promptly.

Genital herpes is not so common as cold sores of the lip, but it is certainly abundant. Since physicians are not required to report genital herpes as they are syphilis and gonorrhea, estimates of the frequency are somewhat uncertain, but the figure of 300,000 new cases a year in the United States today is often quoted. Virtually unknown a few years ago, genital herpes is now the number two venereal disease, slightly less common than gonorrhea, but not far behind it and rapidly gaining ground. Public health authorities have come to speak of the recent upsurge of the disease as an *epidemic*.

Furthermore, changing sexual practices are affecting the nature of the disease. Herpes outbreaks in and around the anus are now observed increasingly in both men and women. And, presumably reflecting the frequency of oral sex, herpes-1 virus now accounts for some 5 to 10 percent of genital herpes infections. (Presumably the type-2 virus can also infect the mouth, but the prevalence of the type-1 virus makes the reverse course more likely.)

Whereas genital herpes can be a painful, and at times a humiliating, condition, it would not be a major medical problem except for (1) the fact that infants born of infected mothers may be seriously, even fatally infected, and (2) the supposition that genital herpes can lead to cervical cancer.

There is some uncertainty about how the virus is transmitted from mother to child, but two modes are probable. In the first, the fetus is infected well before birth, while it is still in the womb, and the virus causes various disturbances in fetal development. The child that results may be born prematurely (some miscarriages probably occur), and it will likely suffer from fever, jaundice, and encephalitis. The usual herpes sores are observed on the skin and in the mouth and eyes. The internal organs, including the liver, brain, kidney, and so on, may be badly damaged and deformed. The outlook for such children is not good.

In the second mode of infection, the infant does not acquire the virus until during the birth process itself, when he is exposed as he passes through the birth canal. (Some infants are exposed at birth by hospital attendants with active herpes infections, and they experience the same course of disease.) These children generally show the first signs of illness on the fourth to seventh day after birth, beginning with lethargy and loss of appetite. The herpetic skin eruption then appears, followed by more serious signs of internal infection, such as fever, jaundice, and convulsions. The condition rapidly worsens, and about half the infected infants die. Many of the rest are permanently impaired (with blindness, mental retardation, or other serious abnormality). Yet, some few infants experience only a mild attack of disease, with light fever and a few herpes sores.

The connection between genital herpes and cancer is largely circumstantial: women with genital herpes are far more likely than other women to develop cervical cancer (see CANCER). It is also suspected— and here the evidence is even less good—that genital herpes in men may lead to penile, even prostatic, cancer. (There is also some suspicion that the herpes-1 virus may be involved in certain types of cancer).

There is little doubt about how the herpes virus is spread—by physical contact, either directly or through the agency of utensils and environmental surfaces (though the virus does not survive long outside the body). Viruses are emitted from typical herpes sores, and they are also contained in saliva and genital secretions even when no sores are present; hence, infected persons can act as carriers when the disease is quiescent. Usually the virus enters the body by way of the mucous membranes, but it can do so through breaks in the skin. Kissing and sexual relations are the primary activities by which the virus is spread, but it can be acquired through other physical contact, such as wrestling, and a person may carry it to his eyes on his own fingers.

The primary infection is the result of virus multiplication soon after the virus has entered the body. Fever and the other generalized reactions indicate that there is a degree of *viremia* at this time. Presumably the initial infection is ended by a mobilization of the body's defenses, *interferon*, *antibodies*, and scavenger cells.

The puzzling, all but unique (see, however, SLOW VIRUS DISEASE), aspect of herpes infections is the recurrence. Most virus infections are hit-and-run affairs that leave at least a degree of immunity behind them. (Repeated colds are often invasions by fresh cold viruses.) One model for this behavior of the herpes virus is that of the CHICKEN POX virus, which when immunity wanes returns (only once, however) to cause shingles. Before its reemergence, the chicken pox virus—which, it turns out, is related to the herpes virus—can be found in cells of the nervous system. There is now good evidence that the herpes virus, too, waits in nerve cells between its recurrent attacks.

Exactly what permits the herpes virus to persist in nerve cells and repeatedly venture out to create herpes sores even in the face of antibodies against the virus is not clear. In *tissue cultures* it is noted that herpes-infected cells can merge with other, uninfected cells, presumably permitting the virus to move into the new cells without encountering the antibodies in the surrounding fluids. Ultimately, however, it is probably the presence of antibodies that causes the recurrent attacks to be so circumscribed, compared to the initial infection. The fact that recurrent attacks are initiated by such traumatic events as fevers or hormonal changes suggests that such events act as triggering mechanisms, releasing the virus from some constraints it experiences while held within the nerve cells.

Under ordinary circumstances, the diagnosis of herpes infections is quite straightforward; the symptoms are clear enough, and no other disease acts quite the same way. Nevertheless, there are times when an absolutely accurate judgment is called for—this is certainly the case with pregnant women—and then laboratory identification of the virus may be necessary.

For laboratory diagnosis a number of procedures are available. One is a simple skin test (like the tuberculin test for tuberculosis), in which killed viruses are placed under the skin and the degree of reaction is observed. An intense reaction indicates a current or recent infection. Another method is to examine specially stained material from the sores under the microscope—if the sores are herpetic, certain large cells are clearly visible. Samples of infected tissue can be examined for herpes viruses by a procedure utilizing fluorescent antibodies, or the samples can be injected into tissue cultures, hens' eggs, or small laboratory animals to see if characteristic signs of infection appear. In cases of herpes encephalitis or meningitis, it may be difficult to obtain tissue specimens for examination except on autopsy. In any suspected instances of primary herpes, however, *serologic tests* for antibodies can be run early and late in the infection to see if a rise of antibodies has occurred.

What to do about herpes infections is a serious medical problem. To a considerable extent the choice of therapy depends on the nature and severity of each particular case. The more serious forms, including herpetic encephalitis and meningitis, eczema herpeticum, and generalized herpes of the newborn, require hospitalization and the most careful medical attention. *Gamma globulin* and herpes *immune globulin* may be helpful here. But even with the best of care, death has not always been avoidable in these cases. Now, medical researchers working with the drug vidarabine have had considerable success in treating victims of herpes encephalitis.

Primary attacks of the more conventional kind also should be looked at by the physician—herpes of the eye is especially dangerous. In infants and very young children, stomatitis may interfere even with liquid intake, and to prevent dehydration in severe cases liquids may be provided intravenously. Recurrent herpes is usually not serious enough to call for medical assistance, though recurrent herpes in the eye must be carefully watched for signs of corneal involvement. Drying agents, such as alcohol, are sometimes applied to blistered areas, and disinfectants may limit their extent. The use of X rays to dry up local sores is not recommended, and most authorities advise the use of antibiotics only when secondary, bacterial infections are known to be present.

The frequency of attacks can often be controlled by careful avoidance of triggering stimuli, such as sunlight and particular foods and drugs.

When emotional factors seem to produce repeated attacks, psycho-therapy may be called for.

Women with recurrent genital herpes clearly have special problems. When outbreaks occur at or near the conclusion of pregnancy, the physician may suggest that the child be delivered by Caesarean section to avoid infection during birth. The possibility that intrauterine infection has already occurred cannot be ruled out in such cases—even less so when herpes has erupted early in pregnancy—and abortions have been recommended on such grounds. To aid in the early detection of cervical cancer, it is recommended that women with genital herpes have yearly gynecological examinations.

A number of special treatments for herpes have been introduced in recent years, some of doubtful value. Because the onset of recurrent herpes may to some extent be under the control of emotional factors, suggestibility plays a role in herpes therapy—if the patient is convinced that a particular regimen may prevent attacks, their frequency may actually be reduced.

One recently introduced treatment—of questionable value—is the use of frequent SMALLPOX vaccinations, which are themselves not without medical risk. This process is said to act by stimulating the body's immunity system, and a number of more justified methods of immunotherapy for herpes are now being studied. One involves the use of an antituberculosis vaccine, BCG; others include the use of supposed innumotherapeutic drugs, levamisole and inosiplex.

For a time authorities favored the employment of a light-sensitive dye (neutral red or proflavine) followed by a 15-minute exposure to ultraviolet light. As a result of this treatment the frequency of recurrences was said to be cut in half. The method is no longer used routinely, however, because in laboratory studies it was found to render supposedly inactivated herpes viruses capable of transforming normal cells into cancer cells.

One drug that is already known to be effective against herpes viruses and that has been approved for limited use is idoxuridine. This substance can be applied only to the cornea, however (or employed topically on the skin); it it too toxic for internal use. The success of vidarabine in treating herpes encephalitis on a trial basis has been referred to above. A number of other new drugs have proved successful in tests and are also now approaching the stage where they may be made available for human use. Included in this group are isoprinosine, levamisole, ribavirin, vidarabine, and phosphonoacetic acid. (Ribavirin and vidarabine have now been found to cause birth defects in experimental animals, however, and that may limit their use.) Out of the large array of antiherpes drugs now being tested, it does not seem too much to hope that at least one will prove to be safe and effective.

Research is also under way on antiherpes vaccines, and several experimental ones have already been prepared. There are two problems with the use of such vaccines, however. One is the matter of recurrent infection. It seems unlikely that vaccination after the initial attack would prevent the recurrent outbreaks, since the original infection—usually a more potent generator of antibodies than vaccination is—itself fails to do so. The only hope, then, is that vaccination before the initial infection would prevent it as well as the recurrent attacks. This has yet to be determined.   •

A potentially even more serious objection to the use of herpes vaccines is the strong possibility that herpes viruses can cause cancer. If this is indeed the case, injecting even weakened or inactivated viruses, which vaccines are composed of, would be unwise until it was definitely established that these could not cause cancer. Nevertheless, in spite of such legitimate concerns, there is still hope that herpes vaccines can be developed, and the disease is serious enough and common enough to justify the effort involved.

The particles of the herpes virus are large, 150 to 200 nanometers in diameter (six to eight millionths of an inch), and physically identical—or nearly so—with those of the chicken pox virus. The inner core contains *DNA* within an *icosahedral* structure of protein subunits. The *outer envelope* consists of several layers of membrane, formed in large part of cellular material, which the virus picks up as it leaves the cell.

The virus can be grown in the corneas of rabbits and guinea pigs, and some strains produce generalized infections in these animals. Suckling mice undergo a rapidly fatal infection following injection. Characteristic pocks are produced when the virus is grown on the membranes of hens' eggs. A wide variety of tissue cultures is susceptible to the virus, most developing characteristic and clearly visible signs of infection.

Reactions with antibodies permit the differentiation of the two otherwise identical types. Antibody studies also show family resemblances to the chicken pox virus and the cytomegalovirus (see CYTOMEGALO-VIRUS INFECTION), as well as to a number of herpes viruses of animals.

HERPES SIMPLEX. See HERPES.

HERPES ZOSTER. See SHINGLES.

HODGKIN'S DISEASE. See CANCER.

HYDROPHOBIA. See RABIES.

INFANTILE PARALYSIS. See POLIO.

INFECTIOUS HEPATITIS (INFECTIOUS JAUNDICE). See
HEPATITIS.

INFECTIOUS MONONUCLEOSIS. See MONONUCLEOSIS.

INFECTIOUS PAROTITIS. See MUMPS.

INFLUENZA (FLU). Primarily a RESPIRATORY INFECTION, but with
high fever and other symptoms of generalized illness, influenza is an
epidemic disease, highly variable in severity. Whereas minor and somewhat restricted outbreaks occur somewhere every year, great *pandemics*
sweep virtually the entire world at 10- to 12-year intervals. The virus, for
reasons that are still not fully understood, is itself quite variable, with the
result that new strains continually find a foothold in populations that are
largely immune to the old strains. The great variation in severity of the
disease, which is probably traceable to changes in the virus, means that
many more fatalities occur in some outbreaks than others. The worst
epidemic in this respect—possibly the worst epidemic of any disease in
world history—is the great pandemic of 1918/19, which took 20 million
lives around the world. Vaccines against influenza are available, but their
use has been a matter of controversy for a long time, and usually they are
given only to the elderly or to others considered to be especially
vulnerable to the disease. In 1976 the United States government began
—and ultimately had to call off—a highly controversial campaign
to vaccinate the entire country against the so-called swine flu, presumed
to be a variant of the virus that had caused the pandemic of 1918. A drug,
amantadine, also is available as a protective measure, but it is not widely
used.

The name of the disease is borrowed from the Italian, in which
language it means "influence," and it is variously said to refer to the
influence of the cold weather or of the stars on the onset of the disease—in
either case, reflecting a seasonal incidence; whereas cases can occur at
any time, epidemics tend to occur in winter, the traditional "flu season."
The disease seems to have been described by Hippocrates in the 5th

century B.C., but the first true recognition of it comes much later. The first description in English is that of the British physician John Huxham in 1743.

Until the late 19th century influenza was thought to be spread simply by the wind, but in 1892 Richard Pfeiffer, a German bacteriologist, attributed the disease to a bacillus he discovered, Hemophilus influenzae. In the epidemic of 1918, however, it was determined that this bacillus was but a contributory agent, with the main cause most likely a virus. In 1931 a swine influenza virus was discovered, and in 1933 the first human flu virus was isolated in London. (Key to success in isolation of the virus was transmission of the disease to ferrets, then mice.) In 1940 a second human virus, designated the influenza B virus, was found—the London virus was then known as the A virus—and in time a C virus also was isolated. Since that time, influenza A has proved to be the most common, and the most variable—the swine viruses are of this type, and those that cause most human epidemics are, as well. The B viruses appear less frequently, and the outbreaks tend to be of limited extent. The C virus is the least troublesome of the three: the illness it causes is mild, and cases are infrequent and sporadic.

Typically, a case of the flu—especially the A variety; the B, like the C, is milder—begins abruptly, after an *incubation period* of a day or two, with a sharp chill, fatigue, and a general achiness. The temperature quickly rises to 101° F to 104° F and then levels off. The symptoms, which last about three days—two to five days is the usual range—are general and not limited to the region of the nose and throat, though some nasal congestion and a ''raw'' throat and dry cough are common. Headache, lassitude, muscle pain, and depression are almost invariably present, and the patient is likely to be prostrated from the beginning. Intestinal disturbances, such as vomiting and diarrhea, however, are rare; the so-called stomach flu is a form of GASTROENTERITIS, rather than a true influenza. THE COMMON COLD is not always clearly distinguishable from flu by the symptoms alone, and the two are often confused. But a cold is generally more localized—severe nasal congestion and copious nasal discharge are the rule with a cold rather than the exception, and the adult cold-sufferer generally does not run a fever.

With young persons, recovery from flu usually occurs rapidly after the fifth day; with the elderly, weakness is likely to persist for some time. With patients at any age, if recovery has not at least begun in five days, it is probably because complications have arisen. These are likely to be infections of the lower respiratory tract, bronchitis, or pneumonia. Generally these are due to secondary invasions by bacteria (such as

Hemophilus influenzae), but in some cases the virus alone is the culprit. Pneumonia is the most serious problem: it is often fatal, especially with patients who are suffering from preexisting heart disease or lung disorders, such as emphysema. For reasons that are not clear, the percentage of cases showing viral pneumonia (often unaccompanied by bacterial invasion) rises during epidemics. This was particularly true of the 1918 pandemic, in which deaths from this complication were unusually high among young adult males. At the same time, in every epidemic there are a great many instances of *inapparent infection*, in which the patient experiences no illness at all or only a slight, transient discomfort in the nose and throat.

The mode of transmission of the disease is clear enough—virus particles are emitted in moist droplets when the patient coughs or sneezes (even ordinary exhaling may be enough), and these droplets remain in the air or dry to an infectious dust. The virus is then inhaled, and the disease process begins in the nose and throat. The localized symptoms (nasal irritation, sore throat, and cough) are the rather obvious result of damage to the cells of the mucous membranes. The more generalized symptoms—fever, headache, lassitude, and muscular aches and pains—are thought to be either a bodily response to the large amounts of cell debris resulting from the destructive action of the virus, or a sensitivity reaction—something like an allergic reaction—brought about by exposure to an *antigen* previously encountered, in this case the virus. Possibly both processes contribute.

The epidemiological patterns of influenza are interesting. Both the A and B viruses attack in series of closely spaced, epidemic waves, followed by a breathing space in which little disease is found. The major A epidemics, each comprised of several waves, tend to occur at two- to three-year intervals; the B epidemics at four- to six-year intervals. In an A epidemic, virtually all elements of the population are hit to an equal extent, though the elderly may be the most seriously affected by the disease. The B epidemics make themselves felt most in institutions, particularly schools, military camps, and nursing homes. In milder epidemics only about 10 percent of the population actually becomes ill; in severe ones, up to 40 percent.

Both forms of the virus vary slightly between epidemics, a process referred to as antigenic "drift," and this is one reason repeated epidemics are possible in the same area—people immune to the old virus strains are only partially so to the new one. The A virus, in addition, undergoes a major antigenic change, or "shift," every 10 or 12 years, producing a quite different strain and one that the population at large is not immune to.

It is the appearance of these essentially new variants of the A virus that
leads to the great pandemics that characterize the disease.

Three such major antigenic shifts have been observed since the first A
strain was isolated in 1933. The first new form, designated A_1 (or
A-prime), appeared in 1946; the second, A_2, in 1957—the A_2 disease
was called Asian flu. The third new form, which first showed up in 1968,
was designated A/Hong Kong, or Hong Kong flu. Since then, a number
of minor variants of the Hong Kong virus have come in succession:
A/England in 1972, A/Port Chalmers (New Zealand) in 1973, A/Scotland
in 1974, and A/Victoria (Australia) in 1975.

This matter of antigenic "drift" and "shift" is all but unique among
viruses, and there is no full explanation for it. Part of the answer seems to
be that the *nucleic acid* of the virus—in effect, the virus genes—is in a
number of different pieces, and this makes possible the exchange of
pieces—genes—between slightly different viruses when they invade the
same cell simultaneously. Another factor probably involved is the ability
of the human virus to invade pigs and possibly other animals (the virus of
1918 is thought to have settled in swine), with a partial exchange of genes
occurring between the viruses of human origin and the normal viruses of
the animal hosts.

There are conflicting hypotheses as to whether the antigenic changes
that occur are continuous, with an endless chain of new forms appearing,
or whether they are cyclical, with a return of old forms after a number of
years. The presence in very old persons of *antibodies* to some of the new
variants that appear suggests that such persons had already been exposed
to these forms in their youth. Certainly this argues in favor of the cyclical
hypothesis, but scientists will not be really sure until one of the variants
that has been isolated in recent years and fully characterized does
reappear. Whatever the cause of the variant forms, their success in
competing with the old forms and quickly supplanting them is easily
understood: it is because so much of the population is not resistant to
them, as it is to the older forms.

The diagnosis of influenza is generally made on the basis of clinical
symptoms alone—the high fever, for example, which differentiates it
from the common cold—but laboratory diagnosis is often conducted for
public health reasons, especially when the appearance of a new strain of
virus is suspected. For testing, viruses are gathered by throat swabs and
grown in eggs or *tissue cultures* of monkey kidney cells. The virus is
easily detected in samples by its ability to cause red blood cells to
agglutinate, or stick together. A positive diagnosis of influenza can also

be made without isolating the virus if a fourfold rise in antibodies in the blood is found by *serologic tests*.

Treatment of the disease consists chiefly in trying to reduce fever and cough; hence, aspirin, cough syrups, and warm liquids are often given. Antibiotics are not employed unless bacterial complications appear. No specific drugs are available for treatment once the disease is under way, but amantadine can be employed as a preventive—a dose is given at the first sign of infection in the community. This method of combating the disease has never become popular, however, probably because the FDA has required clinical testing of the drug against each new strain of the virus that appears, a requirement that is not made for vaccines. Hence, the manufacturer has been unable to advertise the drug as effective against new strains.

Other, still experimental drugs have shown activity against the flu virus in laboratory tests. One of the most studied of these is the substance ribavirin. This material has had mixed success in clinical tests carried out during influenza outbreaks, and its use in human beings appears to be limited because the drug has caused birth defects when given to pregnant laboratory animals. Another drug that seems effective in laboratory tests is levamisole, a drug that acts by stimulating the immunity system.

Killed-virus vaccines are the chief method of prevention, but their effectiveness is somewhat limited (about a 70 percent reduction of disease is observed in vaccinated groups), and the duration of protection is brief, perhaps not more than a year or two. Some promising work has been done on *live-virus vaccines*, which are sprayed directly into the nose or throat, and these have reportedly found some use in Eastern Europe.

The first flu vaccine was prepared in 1943 and successfully used on United States servicemen in 1945. When the new A1 strain appeared a year later, however, the vaccine proved ineffective against it, and a new vaccine had to be developed. Since then authorities have tried to keep one step ahead of the virus, incorporating new strains into the vaccine as soon - as they appear. To this end, the World Health Organization maintains reference laboratories in various parts of the world, which monitor the viruses circulating in the nearby populations.

Unfortunately, when a major antigenic shift in the virus occurs, the new virus is likely to take over very quickly, and sweep around the world before enough new vaccine can be readied to stop it. This happened in 1957 with the Asian flu and again in 1968 with the Hong Kong variety. In the 1968 epidemic up to 50 million Americans were affected, and there were an estimated 30,000 deaths.

In light of the various drawbacks associated with the flu vaccines, they are usually used on a routine basis only for patients in greatest danger from the disease—older persons and those with HEART DISEASE, DIABETES, and chest conditions. Also, military personnel are vaccinated regularly, as are health workers who may be frequently exposed to the virus, but the members of the general public are simply permitted to seek vaccination at their own discretion.

The United States' first (and possibly its last) departure from this procedure came in 1976 when a mass vaccination campaign, one designed to immunize the entire population, was undertaken in response to the appearance of a new virus variant. The new virus, which showed up at Fort Dix, New Jersey, early in the year, proved to be related to swine virus—it was officially dubbed A/New Jersey, unofficially swine flu. An uncertain number of recruits had been infected: a "handful" of cases were actually detected, but many more could have occurred. There was one confirmed death.

Public Health officials were doubly alarmed by the appearance of the new virus. It was nearly time for the next expected shift in the virus to occur, and if this were the new variant it might very quickly begin its march around the world. Furthermore, the relationship of the new virus to the swine virus suggested in turn a relation to the deadly flu virus of 1918, a prospect that was particularly frightening.

It was in response to what at first appeared to be virtually unanimous recommendations from the medical community that President Gerald Ford acted to begin a $135 million program to produce a swine flu vaccine and vaccinate every American before the 1976/77 flu season would get under way. Although several other countries at once elected to follow the lead of the United States, most chose instead to prepare and stockpile vaccine against an outbreak, should one occur. In the United States, however, it was argued that the long time needed to vaccinate 200 million people would make such an approach ineffective.

No sooner was the President's program announced than it came under attack: first, on the grounds that it was politically motivated—the President was then in the early stages of an election campaign—and second, on the score that the vaccine was unlikely to be effective and might well be dangerous. Indeed, the program ran into trouble from the beginning. To start with, the drug makers scheduled to produce the vaccine claimed to have difficulties in procuring insurance against liability for failures of the vaccine, and Congress had to vote to take over such liability. Then, one of the makers proceeded to turn out two million doses of the wrong vaccine. Next, clinical testing showed that though the vaccine was safe and effective for adults (even this conclusion was disputed by some), it was less of both for children.

Nevertheless, with these difficulties behind it, the nationwide vaccination campaign began in October 1976 ("Roll Up Your Sleeve, America"). Adults between the ages of 18 and 60 received the swine flu vaccine alone. (A special children's vaccine was still under development.) The elderly and those at special risk were given a bivalent vaccine, which also contained the A/Victoria virus, still considered a threat.

Again trouble appeared. In mid-October three elderly persons in Philadelphia, who had been vaccinated within an hour of one another from the same lot of vaccine, died suddenly and unexpectedly. When this and a number of other early deaths among elderly vaccinees came to light, vaccination was suspended. Yet, autopsy showed all deaths to be due to other causes, and statistical analyses revealed that their number was not greater than what would have been expected without vaccination. Although the vaccination program was resumed, much of the public was now suspicious, and the rate of vaccination remained low.

In December, the program again was suspended when it was observed that an unexpectedly large number of cases of an obscure neurological disease, the GUILLAIN-BARRÉ SYNDROME, were occurring among those vaccinated. Although the number of cases of Guillain-Barré was not large—ultimately close to 500 were found in the country, about half among the 50 million who had been vaccinated—still it was estimated that those who had been vaccinated were 7.5 times as likely to develop the disease (it produces temporary paralysis) as those who had not.

For the young adult public, vaccination was not now resumed. Only a few isolated cases of swine flu had appeared since the original outbreak, and some authorities had concluded that the virus did not pass easily from person to person (but moved mainly from swine to human beings). For the elderly, however, vaccination with the bivalent vaccine was resumed. The A/Victoria virus was thought to be enough of a danger to such persons to warrant the very slight risk of Guillain-Barré syndrome. (There was no A/Victoria vaccine available that had not been mixed with the swine flu material.)

In retrospect it seems clear that a courageous, but probably misguided, effort had been made to avoid a major medical catastrophe. The massive vaccination campaign to forestall the new virus before it was clearly shown to be a threat was probably a mistake. The risk associated with any mass vaccination is such that it is better not undertaken unless there is a clear and present danger. In the future, it seems likely that Public Health officials will continue their policy of monitoring flu viruses in the field, preparing vaccines against new strains as they appear, and vaccinating only when outbreaks actually occur.

The influenza virus itself—which is, of course, ultimately responsible for the disease—consists of particles that are roughly spherical (*icosahedral*), with a diameter of about 100 nanometers (four millionths of an inch). Forming the surface of the particles is an *outer envelope* covered with spikes. Inside is the single-stranded RNA (in eight separate segments) and associated protein. These inner materials form a *helix* about 10 nanometers in diameter, which is wound into a compact shape. Often accompanying the spherical particles are filamentlike structures up to 10 times as long.

Although the particles of the three different viruses A, B, and C look the same under the electron microscope, they are not identical, as can be shown by studies with antibodies. These are largely carried out with a so-called soluble antigen, which is produced by the virus in infected cells and which can easily be separated from the virus particles. The different strains of the various types are also detected by antibody studies—in this case, advantage is taken of the ability of the virus particles to cause red cells to agglutinate. Antibodies that are especially adapted to the surface peculiarities of each separate strain prevent only those strains and no others from agglutinating cells.

JAPANESE ENCEPHALITIS (JAPANESE B ENCEPHALITIS). See ST. LOUIS ENCEPHALITIS.

JAUNDICE. See HEPATITIS.

JUVENILE RHEUMATOID ARTHRITIS. See ARTHRITIS.

KOREAN HEMORRHAGIC FEVER. See HEMORRHAGIC FEVER.

KURU. A chronic, always fatal, disease caused by degeneration of the brain, kuru is limited to the Fore people, a tribe of New Guinea cannibals. The word "kuru" means trembling, or shaking, and this is the most prominent early symptom of the disease. As the illness proceeds, movements become spastic and tortured, the eyes cross, and the patient may be swept by bouts of uncontrolled laughing or weeping. Death occurs after about two years. A virus of unusual properties is thought to be the cause of kuru, and the disorder is generally classed as a SLOW VIRUS DISEASE.

What is known about the epidemiology of kuru among the Fore is chiefly due to the work of D. Carleton Gajdusek, now at the National Institutes of Health, who spent a year with the primitive tribe in the late 1950s—in 1976 Gajdusek shared in the Nobel Prize in Medicine for his work on kuru. The disease has been *epidemic* among the Fore for some time, though other neighboring tribes did not experience it—suggesting a hereditary element in the disorder. But after studying the customs of the tribe, Gajdusek concluded that the disease was transmitted by a ritual handling and eating of the brains of dead relatives—themselves victims of the disease—as a sign of respect. Later, in 1963, Gajdusek provided evidence that kuru is infectious by injecting material from the brains of kuru victims into chimpanzees, who then died of the disease in two to three years.

Now, cannibalism has been abandoned by the Fore, and kuru too is on the wane. Nonetheless, it may be some time before the disease disappears altogether. Because it has a very long *incubation period*—possibly up to 20 years—many people already infected may not yet show signs of the disease.

In a rather curious footnote to the story of kuru among the Fore, it has been suggested, based on the condition of skeletons, that Neanderthal man practiced a similar rite, eating (or at least removing) the brains of deceased relatives. Possibly, then—and this, of course, is sheer speculation—the disappearance of Neanderthal man might have been brought about by kuru or a similar disease.

The symptoms of kuru are caused by wholesale destruction of nerve cells in the brain. This is shown by microscopic examination of the brain on autopsy, which reveals a peculiar spongy look of the diseased tissue. This spongy appearance is also found in the brains of victims of another rare disorder, CREUTZFELDT-JAKOB DISEASE. And two animal diseases, scrapie (a disorder of sheep) and transmissible mink encephalopathy, produce the same effect.

Because of this similarity, these diseases are suspected of being caused by similar agents. Although such agents might well be viruses—and the diseases behave in many ways like other slow virus diseases—careful studies have revealed many unusual properties of these materials. Chemically, physically, and biologically, they do not act like virus particles. As a result, some authorities have come to believe that these agents represent an entirely new class of infective agent, a new kind of microorganism.

KYASANUR FOREST DISEASE. See HEMORRHAGIC FEVER.

LA CROSSE ENCEPHALITIS. See CALIFORNIA ENCEPHALITIS.

LASSA FEVER. A severe, almost always fatal, illness that occurs in East Africa, Lassa fever is notable because it is wildly contagious in hospitals and laboratories. The most damaging effect is hemorrhaging of the internal organs (see HEMORRHAGIC FEVER); death often occurs following kidney failure. The natural host of the virus is an African rat. In nature, the viruses are suspected of spreading to human beings by way of dried dusts from rat urine and feces; in institutions, however, the virus has been known to spread via cuts or nicks in the skin. It may also be airborne. Research on the virus is now conducted only in laboratories with special containment equipment, which permits the virus to be handled by remote control.

The virus first came to light in 1969 when three missionary nurses in a hospital in Lassa, Nigeria, contracted fatal cases of the disease. Research on the virus at Yale University, which began at this time, was stopped abruptly when several research workers acquired the disease, one fatally. Between 1969 and 1972 epidemics occurred in two other countries, Liberia and Sierra Leone, and surveys suggest that the virus has appeared elsewhere in East Africa but gone unrecognized. The fatality rate of hospitalized patients has been high—42 percent—and in all some 14 nurses and a physician have been infected while caring for patients.

Symptoms begin with fever, chills, headache, and joint aches and pains. A temporary remission may occur after a day or two, but soon the fever returns, climbing even higher. (Temperatures of 107°F have been recorded.) At this time ulcerous sores appear in the throat, and small areas of hemorrhaging occur in the skin, leaving purplish marks. Soon signs of kidney failure are noted, as urine output decreases and finally ceases entirely. Autopsy of fatal cases reveals extensive internal hemorrhaging, with heavy damage to the kidney, liver, and lungs.

The only effective therapy is the use of *immune serum* drawn from patients convalescent from the disease. There is no drug to combat the virus, and vaccines have not been developed.

Extensive field study of bats and rodents in areas where the disease occurs in Africa revealed viruses only in one species of rat, Mastomys natalensis, which lives in the wild as well as in human dwellings. The best way to limit the spread of the virus seems to be by control of the rat host. This can be accomplished effectively by rat poisons, such as warfarin.

The virus is related to the LYMPHOCYTIC CHORIOMENINGITIS virus and to the Machupo and Junin viruses, which cause hemorrhagic fever. These viruses all infect bats or rodents, often for long periods without producing acute signs of disease, and they are transmitted to man by way of the animals' excreta. They thus differ from the arboviruses (see ARBOVIRUS DISEASE), which by definition are transmitted by the bites of insects or other arthropods. It has been proposed, therefore, that the Lassa fever and related viruses be classed as a separate group—to be referred to as arenaviruses.

LCM. See LYMPHOCYTIC CHORIOMENINGITIS.

LEUKEMIA. See CANCER.

LOUPING ILL. See TICK-BORNE ENCEPHALITIS.

LUPUS. See SYSTEMIC LUPUS ERYTHEMATOSUS.

LYME ARTHRITIS. See ARTHRITIS.

LYMPHOCYTIC CHORIOMENINGITIS (LCM). A disease acquired from mice, hamsters, and guinea pigs, lymphocytic choriomeningitis either is flu-like or produces a type of MENINGITIS. It is often mild, sometimes more serious, but rarely fatal. In mice the disease takes the form of a persistent but low-grade infection, which may be related to the so-called SLOW VIRUS DISEASES of man.

The name, lymphocytic choriomeningitis, is derived from a commonly observed effect of the disease, the invasion by white blood cells, lymphocytes, of several membranes associated with the brain, the choroid plexuses and the meninges. The course of the disease is highly variable. After an *incubation period* of one to three weeks, flu-like symptoms generally appear, consisting of fever, headache, cough, sore throat, and muscle aches and pains. In a majority of cases, this is all that happens. But after a period of improvement of about a week, there may be a return of fever, along with signs of meningitis, namely headache and a stiff neck. Occasionally drowsiness or mild agitation, signs of EN-CEPHALITIS, are observed, and the disease has been known to cause inflammation of the salivary glands of the jaws, thereby imitating MUMPS. In the few fatal cases that have occurred, extensive damage to the central nervous system has been found on autopsy.

Many cases of human lymphocytic choriomeningitis have been acquired from wild mice—the virus is thought to spread in dusts from dried mouse urine and feces. Also, laboratory personnel are easily infected from colonies of mice and hamsters. Pet owners, too, are susceptible. In 1974 an epidemic in upper New York State caused by the sale of infected hamsters as pets mounted to 57 cases.

There is no cure for choriomeningitis, and no vaccine has been developed. Treatment, of course, is dependent on the nature and severity of the symptoms—often bed rest is sufficient, but hospitalization is required in more serious cases. Control is achieved in homes by rodent eradication or removal of infected pets. Suppliers of pets and laboratory animals should screen all animals sold, but because many animals are capable of carrying the virus without showing signs of illness, screening is difficult and must be carried out by laboratory testing.

In human patients laboratory diagnosis of lymphocytic choriomeningitis is achieved by isolation of the virus from cerebrospinal fluid, blood, or material from throat swabs. For testing, samples are injected into uninfected mice, in which they produce symptoms of the disease. The virus can also be detected in patients by rises in blood *antibodies* observed by *serologic tests*. Viruses are found in persistently infected mice, who do not show signs of infection, by injection into other mice, known not to be infected.

The state of persistent infection in mice is reached when unborn mice pick up the virus from their mothers in utero or immediately after birth. In such mice the viruses multiply and remain in the body throughout the animals' lifetime, apparently because certain classes of antibodies do not form. (The virus is already present before the antibody system matures and is not recognized as being alien to the body.) Nevertheless, these mice do not have normal life expectancies and generally die of disturbances reminiscent of human CONNECTIVE TISSUE DISEASE. Although there is no evidence of persistent human infections with lymphocytic choriomeningitis virus, the unusual circumstance that the virus remains in the animal for long periods suggests a resemblance to the "slow" virus diseases.

The virus is an *RNA* virus of large, and variable, size (50 to over 300 nanometers in diameter, or 2 to 12 millionths of an inch). The particles carry an *outer envelope* and somewhat resemble the arboviruses (see ARBOVIRUS DISEASE). But the virus is most closely related to the LASSA FEVER virus and the HEMORRHAGIC FEVER viruses of the Tacaribe group. This relationship is shown by antibody studies, by the fact that all the viruses infect rodents (perhaps chronically) and are carried to man by rodent excreta, and by the irregular nature of the virus particles, each of which is composed of a number of granules, about 20 nanometers in diameter (the size of many small viruses). This last property has given the group the name arenaviruses, "arena-" being a Latin root meaning "sandy," a reference to the granularity of the particles.

MARBURG DISEASE (GREEN MONKEY DISEASE). A deadly disorder characterized by high fever and hemorrhaging, Marburg disease was first observed in 1967 in the West German town of Marburg, among laboratory workers handling organs from African green monkeys. The disease has since been found to occur naturally in Africa, but it is not clear how widespread it is, or how long a history it has had. In 1975 three cases (one fatal) appeared in South Africa, and in 1976 an epidemic in Central Africa took some 320 lives.

A type of HEMORRHAGIC FEVER, Marburg disease generally begins with high fever, headache, and vomiting. External hemorrhaging soon ensues, and internal bleeding, with extensive damage to the liver and kidney, is observed on autopsy. Death rates are high—30 to 50 percent.

Like the similar LASSA FEVER, the disease spreads readily in hospitals and laboratories. In addition to those infected in the Marburg outbreak, a scientist in a British military research center contracted the disease in 1976. Infection has resulted from nicks in the skin and contact with infected blood. The virus may also be spread by dusts in the air.

Nobody knows how the disease is transmitted in Africa. If the virus behaves like the Lassa fever virus, it may be carried in dusts from dried monkey urine and feces, but possibly it is transmitted by insects as the arboviruses are (see ARBOVIRUS DISEASE). The virus itself has not yet been characterized.

There is no treatment for Marburg disease, but it is hoped that *immune serum* prepared from the blood of recovered victims of the disease will aid others in fighting it. Strict isolation of patients and great care in handling contaminated material are required.

MAYORO VIRUS INFECTION. See DENGUE.

MEASLES (RUBEOLA, MORBILLI). Common, or "red," measles is a virus disease that combines the symptoms of a cold—runny nose, sore throat, and cough—with a reddish skin rash. It is more severe than GERMAN MEASLES, and complications, including pneumonia and a sometimes fatal ENCEPHALITIS, do occur, though not commonly.

Measles used to be the most prevalent of all childhood diseases. Indeed, next to the common cold, it was probably the most prevalent of all diseases—virtually everybody in the world experienced it at one time or another. This picture changed dramatically in the 1960s, however, with the introduction of effective vaccines, which cut the number of annual cases in the United States by some 99 percent. Yet, by the late 1970s, vaccination against measles had begun to taper off, and prospects for eliminating the disease completely had begun to wane—regrettably so, because of the small number of fatalities that always occur.

In 1969, it was established that a rare degenerative disease of the nervous system, SUBACUTE SCLEROSING PANENCEPHALITIS, can be a late follow-up of measles infections, often appearing many years later. And there is some evidence, which is hardly conclusive, suggesting that PAGET'S DISEASE OF BONE, and possibly even MULTIPLE SCLEROSIS and SYSTEMIC LUPUS ERYTHEMATOSUS, also may be late sequels to early measles infection.

There is no doubt that measles is a very old disease, although its early history is obscure because the ancients did not clearly distinguish it from SMALLPOX and other disorders producing skin eruptions. It has been suggested that the disease was introduced to Europe in the eighth century by an invasion of the Saracens. Certainly the disease was clearly described in the 9th century by the Arabian Rhazes, who, however, thought it was a mild form of smallpox. In Europe the distinction between these diseases seems first to have been made in print in 1553 by a Sicilian named Ingrassia, but this distinction probably was not made commonly until the 17th century, when it was reaffirmed by the great English physician Sydenham.

In the 18th century large-scale *epidemics* occurred of a particularly virulent form of the disease known as black measles, which was characterized by bleeding from the mouth, nose, and bowels, and which was often fatal. Although this form continued to appear sporadically in certain parts of the world until well into the 20th century, it now seems to have disappeared completely.

The symptoms of common measles generally begin about 10 days after exposure, with fever and a general sense of discomfort; within a few hours the coldlike symptoms appear, with early sneezing and especially copious nasal discharges. Conjunctivitis, or irritation of the inner lining of the eyelids, is also likely at this time. A day or two later the first signs of the rash appear on the inside of the cheeks. Known as Koplik's spots after their discoverer, an American pediatrician, these characteristic red blotches with white centers (like specks of salt) are a unique and almost invariable sign of measles.

Some 2 days after the appearance of the Koplik's spots, and usually almost exactly 14 days after exposure, the measles rash proper begins.

Typically it starts at the hairline, and over 2 or 3 days slowly works its way downward until it eventually reaches the feet. Unlike the skin eruptions of smallpox and CHICKEN POX, which are pimply or pustular, those of measles are a true rash, consisting of raised, irregular, reddish spots, which may merge to form large welts, particularly over the face and upper body.

Once the rash is fully developed, the patient begins to recover almost at once—unless there are complications. The fever abruptly abates, the conjunctivitis clears up, and the nasal congestion disappears. Only the cough is likely to linger some days longer. At the same time, the rash begins to fade, rarely lasting more than 5 or 6 days in all. As it disappears, the skin takes on a temporary brownish discoloration and small flakes or skin are shed. There is no permanent scarring.

Complications are rare in healthy children today, though they do occur. They are most common among infants and young adults and among children in underdeveloped countries. Most frequent are acute RESPIRATORY INFECTIONS, either bronchitis or pneumonia, and infections of the middle ear. The respiratory infection may be caused by the measles virus itself or by secondary, bacterial invaders, such as streptococci or pneumococci. Its onset is usually signaled by a persistence of high fever after the rash has begun to fade. It is characterized by a deepening, protracted cough and labored, wheezing breathing. Ear infections, which are always bacterial, are marked by earache and sometimes by a discharge. All these complications vary greatly in severity from patient to patient; most often they are mild and of short duration, but they can lead to perforated ear drums and deafness, or a fulminating, fatal pneumonia.

The most serious complication of all is encephalitis, which strikes about one measles patient in a thousand, usually on the fourth day after appearance of the rash. The first symptoms are a resumption of fever and vomiting, accompanied by headache, stiff neck, and drowsiness. Later behavioral changes, coma, and convulsions may occur. In about half the cases, the encephalitis departs rapidly leaving no aftereffects, but in some 15 percent it is fatal, and the rest of the patients show varying degrees of emotional or physical impairment, including spastic conditions, muscular weakness, partial paralysis, and speech difficulties.

Yet there is little doubt that measles today is not the fearsome disease it once was. The hideous black measles of centuries ago is no more, and even before the introduction of vaccines, the death rate from measles had fallen dramatically in the United States and western Europe. Still, the disease remains a serious one in Asia, Africa, and South America, where the fatality rate may reach 10 percent of those stricken. (It is less than 1 percent in the United States today.) Some authorities have taken these facts to mean that the measles virus strain current in Europe and the United States today is a weakened variant—weaker than the ones we used to experience and weaker than those circulating in other parts of the world. Other authorities suggest that the virus has made its home in western Europe for very long periods and that the inhabitants, including those who have migrated to North America, have developed a tolerance for it not shared by the rest of the world. A more likely explanation, however, would seem to be that the population of the developed countries is in a better nutritional state, has better sanitary facilities, and receives better medical care, all of which could increase resistance to the invasions of the virus and also to the bacterial invaders that so often take advantage of the beachheads it opens for them.

Measles is not simply a localized skin disorder. The respiratory distress is one indication of this, but also viruses have been isolated from the blood, urine, and various internal organs, verifying that the infection is a generalized one. The virus almost surely enters the body through the nose and throat (perhaps also through the conjunctival membranes of the eye), after which it begins to multiply in the local lymph glands, enters the bloodstream, and is soon spread around the body, probably continuing to multiply in the white blood cells. Then the virus concentrates its attack on the membranes of the respiratory system and the eyelids, producing the symptoms of a cold and conjunctivitis. Finally comes an attack on the skin, with local multiplication of virus and cell destruction causing the measles rash. An unusual effect of the virus observed in the microscope is the formation of giant cells by the fusion of ordinary body cells. This action undoubtedly plays a part in the tissue damage observed.

Many of the so-called complications, such as bronchitis and pneumonia, simply result from extension of the area of heavy virus attack beyond its usual limitation to the upper respiratory tract. But bacterial invasions in these areas, and in the middle ear, have been amply demonstrated by isolation and identification of the bacterial agents. It is not clear whether measles encephalitis results from destruction in the central nervous system wrought directly by the virus, or whether it is an inflammatory, allergic response to the presence of virus particles or virus-altered cells. Most authorities lean toward the latter view.

Although measles virus is present in the urine, its spread from patient to patient is chiefly by way of droplets admitted to the air by coughing and sneezing. Direct contact with virus-containing saliva or nasal discharges also may bring the disease. The virus does not survive long outside the body, however, and thorough airing of a patient's room is usually enough to decontaminate it.

The disease spreads rapidly among young children, and isolation and quarantine have not been found effective control measures, although children with chronic diseases or malnutrition are often segregated when measles is abroad. The high incidence among children does not indicate any special susceptibility, but rather the usual age of first exposure. When measles has been introduced into isolated island populations, everyone, regardless of age, has been susceptible. Measles was so widespread before the introduction of vaccination that 97 percent of the world's population had experienced an attack by the age of 15 years. Although there may be a few symptomless or *inapparent infections,* they are undoubtedly rare. Almost everyone who contracts measles undergoes the measles rash, and remembers it into adulthood (though there may be confusion between ordinary measles and the German variety). The disease occurs in every part of the world, and in urban areas epidemics typically take place at two-year intervals, or just long enough for a new crop of susceptible children to appear. These epidemics tend to occur in late winter or spring; March and April are the peak months.

The key research that made measles vaccines possible was carried out by John Franklin Enders, the man who first grew polio viruses in *tissue culture,* a feat accomplished in 1949. In 1954, the year Enders and his collaborators received the Nobel Prize for that, he duplicated the work with the measles virus, successfully cultivating it for the first time in cultures of human and chicken cells. Four years later he produced an attenuated virus, suitable for vaccine use.

Two types of measles vaccines are now available: one is *killed-virus vaccines;* the other, live *attenuated vaccines.* The killed virus vaccines are produced by formaldehyde inactivation of culture-grown viruses. Three doses are needed, and protection is not as long-lasting as that produced by the live vaccines. The first of these, which was licensed for general use in 1963, employed the so-called Edmonston strain of viruses, cultivated by Enders. This vaccine gave very good protection after only one injection, but it frequently caused both fever and rash. These side effects could be prevented by simultaneous injection of *gamma globulin* or by the previous use of the killed vaccine. A better vaccine became available in 1965 when a new, further attenuated virus strain, the Schwarz strain, was licensed for vaccine use. It gives nearly as good protection as the Edmonston vaccine, but the incidence of fever and rash is much lower. This vaccine has been widely employed since its introduction. Neither of the live vaccines is effective in children under one year of age because they are still protected by maternal *antibodies* and the vaccine viruses are unable to multiply. Authorities now recommend that vaccination be delayed until the age of 15 months, except when an epidemic is in progress.

Some 60 million children in the United States have been inoculated with these vaccines in the decade following their licensing, and the overall results have been impressive. The number of annual cases has fallen from 4 million to 22,000. Previously there were 400 annual fatalities and 800 children left with serious brain damage; now there is only a "handful" in each category—exact figures are hard to come by.

Yet, in spite of these results, and in spite of the fact that 41 states require measles vaccination before children begin school, the pace of measles vaccination has begun to slow. It is estimated that only 60 percent of school-age children are now protected against measles. And the steadily declining incidence of measles has begun to turn upward. In the winter of 1976/77, the number of cases was running 65 percent above the number for the previous year on a nationwide basis (up from 22,000 to 37,000 cases). Major outbreaks of measles that winter occurred in California, Illinois, Iowa, Missouri, Minnesota, Texas, and Virginia.

Part of the reason for the declining vaccination rate may have been the unpleasant reaction associated with the original vaccine; but now that a milder one is available, the failure to protect children against the disease probably stems chiefly from waning memories of how widespread and how severe the disease used to be—measles has now become one of the "conquered" diseases. But as long as children continue to contract the disease, and some to die of its complications, the disease has hardly been conquered.

It can be, however, almost surely. There is no known wild animal host for the measles virus, and though the virus is present everywhere in the world today, once there are enough protected individuals, it is bound to die out from lack of new susceptible hosts—as seems to be happening with the smallpox virus. One hopeful sign in the United States is the Carter administration's announced intention to see that 90 percent of all youngsters are inoculated by 1979.

Before the measles vaccines were introduced, it was common practice to treat children exposed to the disease with gamma globulin drawn from others recovering from the disease, *immune globulin,* and the practice is still followed when unvaccinated children are exposed. If large doses of immune globulin are given, the disease is completely prevented; if smaller ones are used, a mild case results, and the individual is then fully protected from later infection. This situation is more desirable, of course, so the amount of immune globulin is carefully controlled to bring it about.

Treatment for uncomplicated measles is conventional. Bed rest is mandatory, beginning with the initial fever, which may be treated with aspirin. Cough medicines are not much help usually, though those containing codeine may give some relief. Nose drops do little to halt the nasal discharge. If the eyes are irritated, washing with warm water may help by removing the hardened secretions. Many patients become sensitive to light, and keeping their rooms darkened is advisable.

Antibiotics do nothing to fight the measles virus, and their routine use to prevent complications is not good practice. Some physicians treat all measles patients with antibiotics on the mistaken assumption that it is easier to prevent secondary bacterial infections than to treat them once they have begun. Studies have shown, however, that this is counterproductive in that the antibiotics do not reduce the incidence of secondary infections and that those that develop are drug resistant and harder to treat. Gamma globulin also is sometimes given to prevent complications, and though there is no good evidence that the practice is effective, it surely does no harm.

Complications, of course, call for more dramatic measures. Pneumonia, bronchitis, and middle-ear infections shown to be caused by bacteria are treated at once with antibiotics and generally disappear promptly. When respiratory disease and encephalitis are caused by the measles virus itself, no specific therapy is available. Here careful medical and nursing attention is necessary to assist the patient in every way possible. Liquids may be given intravenously and oxygen may be administered if breathing is obstructed. Encephalitic convulsions may be eased with barbiturates.

It is important to diagnose measles correctly, chiefly in order to avoid confusion with smallpox, which is so serious, and German measles, which can cause major birth defects when it is contracted by pregnant women. Fortunately, diagnosis is simplified by the fact that 90 percent or more of measles patients show Koplik's spots, and these appear in no other disease. The chief source of difficulty is that it is usually especially mild cases of measles that fail to show the spots, and such cases are the ones most easily taken to be German measles or possibly very mild cases of smallpox. Confusion of measles with full-blown smallpox or chicken pox is unlikely because of the pimplelike pocks of those diseases, but in especially mild cases these do not form. Generally, the rash of scarlet fever differs greatly from that of measles, but it, too, may be difficult to distinguish on occasion.

In any case, laboratory diagnosis permits positive identification of the measles virus. The most used method is to look for a marked, rapid increase of antibodies to the virus in the blood during the course of infection, the level of antibodies being determined usually by *serologic tests*. The first blood sample is generally drawn as soon as possible after the rash appears and the second four or five days later; a fourfold rise in antibodies during this period is taken to indicate active infection. Measles viruses themselves can be isolated from the blood, urine, and throat washings of patients and then grown in cell cultures, but the results are somewhat chancy, and this procedure is not used routinely for diagnostic purposes.

The measles virus is rather closely related to viruses that cause distemper in dogs and rinderpest in cattle. Since these animals are, like man, mammalian, and all three species are therefore related, it might seem that these three modern viruses had a common ancestor, which long ago parasitized a mammalian species ancestral to their present animal hosts, and that the three viruses diverged and evolved as their host did. But the three host species are not themselves closely related (were they all higher primates, for example, the situation would be different); and all of them have close relatives that do not harbor similar viruses. Hence the above hypothesis seems unlikely. A more reasonable supposition is based on the rather recent (speaking in evolutionary terms) close association of man, dogs, and cattle. It seems probable that a virus which once parasitized one of these species successfully transferred itself to the others when they began to live near one another. Subsequent adaptation of the virus to its new hosts would then have resulted in the three closely related but not identical viruses we now find.

Like the rinderpest and canine distemper viruses, that of measles is a myxovirus. The particles are roughly spherical, ranging in diameter from 120 to 250 nanometers (five to ten millionths of an inch). The *outer envelope* is covered with small projections, and there is an inner, twisted *helical* core (about 17 nanometers in diameter) made of protein and *RNA*. The virus has been grown in fertile chicken eggs and the brains of young mice, but for most purposes, including vaccine preparation, it is cultivated in cultures of human, monkey, or chicken embryo cells. The monkey is the only animal that has been infected with the virus, and some monkeys in captivity catch measles from their human handlers. In monkeys the disease is mild.

MEASLES, GERMAN. See GERMAN MEASLES.

MENINGITIS. An inflammation of the meninges, the membranes covering the brain and spinal cord, meningitis usually results in fever, headache, vomiting, and stiffness of the neck.

The cause of most cases of meningitis is an infection by the bacterium commonly designated meningococcus. But for a long time it has been known that there also occur cases of "aseptic" (really nonbacterial) meningitis, and these have now been shown to be usually caused by viruses. Although the viruses involved are often not fully identified, those found most frequently are the echo and coxsackie viruses (see COX-SACKIE OR ECHO VIRUS INFECTION), the LYMPHOCYTIC CHORIOMENINGITIS, POLIO, MUMPS, CHICKEN POX, MEASLES, HERPES, and INFLUENZA viruses.

Although meningitis alone is the prevailing disorder in cases of aseptic meningitis, signs of meningitis often occur along with the more usual symptoms of other disorders (especially those whose viruses are listed above as being sometimes responsible for aseptic meningitis). Meningitis and ENCEPHALITIS frequently accompany one another, and meningitis signs are often found among the symptoms resulting from infection by the various encephalitis viruses.

MOLLUSCUM CONTAGIOSUM. A mild, infectious, skin disease that occurs in most areas of the world, molluscum contagiosum (the name means contagious nodules) is characterized by the formation of tiny, soft, wartlike growths. These are pink or white and often possess a central opening that reveals a whitish interior. A milky fluid may be extruded.

Like WARTS, the nodules disappear spontaneously, generally in a matter of months. They can be removed, also like warts, by cauterization.

The disease is spread by direct or indirect contact. Wrestlers and gymnasts are especially likely to get it, but venereal spread is also known. Contamination may be by way of gymnastic or sport equipment, towels, brushes, or household utensils. The sores form at the point of contact, which often is on the face, scalp, trunk, limbs, or genitalia. Rarely do they appear on mucous membranes, however, and supposedly never on the palms of the hands or the soles of the feet.

In its behavior, the molluscum contagiosum virus resembles the warts virus insomuch as it occurs chiefly in the dying cells at the outer portions of the nodule. Structurally, however, the two viruses are very different. Whereas the warts virus is small and compact, the molluscum con-tagiosum virus is large and brick-shaped, with dimensions of 250 by 350 nanometers (10 to 15 millionths of an inch). It is a *DNA* virus that much resembles the pox viruses (see SMALLPOX), and may be a member of that group. It has not been grown in experimental animals or hens' eggs, but it can be cultivated in human cells in *tissue culture*.

MONONUCLEOSIS (INFECTIOUS MONONUCLEOSIS, GLAN-DULAR FEVER).

Mononucleosis, formerly called glandular fever, is a debilitating but rarely fatal disease of teen-agers and young adults; it is especially common among college students and servicemen. Characterized by fever, sore throat, and swelling of the lymph glands, the disease also causes a proliferation of mononuclear white blood cells (from which circumstance the name is drawn). There is now no doubt that the disease is caused by a virus and the virus responsible seems to have been found. Yet, there is no special treatment for the disease, and no vaccine is available.

There is some difference of opinion about the length of the *incubation period*—some authorities place it at four days to two weeks, others at five to seven weeks. At any rate, when they do come, the first symptoms are headache, fever, chills, sore throat, fatigue, and malaise. After a few days the lymph nodes in the neck (and possibly those elsewhere) become swollen. The throat is now raw and red, and the tonsils are inflamed and covered with a whitish fluid, sometimes a grayish membrane. An unpleasant odor from the mouth can often now be noticed. At this time, too, the eyelids may be puffy and swollen and rashes of various kinds may appear on the skin and in the throat.

During this stage of the disease, blood counts reveal the presence of large numbers of the mononuclear white cells. At the same time a unique substance—designated a heterophil *antibody*—is found in the blood. It causes sheep red cells to clump together, or agglutinate, a property that is taken advantage of to produce a diagnostic test for the disease.

The most serious complication is enlargement of the spleen, which occurs in about half the cases; rupture of the spleen has resulted in fatalities. Liver damage, too, is detected fairly often—by liver function tests—and jaundice resembling that of HEPATITIS occasionally occurs. ENCEPHALITIS and MENINGITIS may develop.

Recovery generally takes from a few days to three weeks. Some complaints may persist beyond this time, but relapses and reinfections are rare. Nonetheless, victims of mononucleosis are often easily fatigued and forced to curtail activities for months after apparent recovery. Although the disease is reported to be rare in children, and when it does occur to be quite mild, it is likely that inapparent infections in children are more common than is generally realized.

Mononucleosis is familiarly known as the "kissing disease," and the best scientific evidence supports this assessment of its mode of transmission. The disease is only mildly communicable—scientists have had difficulty transmitting it by throat swabs—but it does seem to be spread by intimate oral contact. Presumably the virus multiplies in the mucous membranes of the throat, then invades the blood, and finally finds its way via the bloodstream to the spleen and liver.

Treatment of the disease depends on the severity of the condition. Often the patient can be cared for at home, but hospitalization may be called for in severe cases. Bed rest, plenty of fluids, and a light diet are desirable. The physician will give careful attention to the throat, and frequent washes with mild salt solution or antiseptics may be employed. Antibiotics are not used routinely. The chief danger is ruptured spleen, and it is the responsibility of the physician to monitor the course of the illness in this respect. Of course, he must watch for signs of hepatitis, meningitis, and encephalitis. (The strict enforcement of bed rest is thought to minimize the risk of such complications.) Since the disease is not considered highly contagious, isolation of the patient is usually not necessary.

Although mononucleosis can sometimes be confused with streptococcal throat infections ("strep throat") or with viral hepatitis, the combination of fever, sore throat, and swollen lymph glands is usually unmistakable evidence of mononucleosis. The raised mononuclear white cell count is confirmatory evidence of mononucleosis, as are several tests based on the presence of the heterophil antibody. Liver function tests may be run to reveal the extent of liver damage.

There is some reason to suspect that the heterophil antibody is itself the virus, or at least a virus product—much as the so-called Australia *antigen* is believed to be a portion of the outer coat of the HEPATITIS B virus particle. For some time, however, scientists have had difficulty isolating the mononucleosis virus. In some cases of mononucleosis, the cytomegalovirus has been implicated (see CYTOMEGALOVIRUS INFECTION), but these instances are thought to be exceptional. More recently, in a sizable number of mononucleosis patients, antibodies have been found to the Epstein-Barr virus, a HERPES virus that is also thought to cause Burkitt's lymphoma (see CANCER). In one recent study of 43 children with mononucleosis, 30 showed clear-cut signs of infection by the Epstein-Barr virus. The relationship between this virus and mononucleosis is not yet fully settled, but it seems safe to assume that the virus is the causative agent. Until the virus is definitely identified and cultivated, there is little hope of developing a vaccine, although if the heterophil antibody is a virus product there is some chance it might be purified and used as a vaccine (as some workers hope to use the Australia antigen as a vaccine against hepatitis B).

MORBILLI. See MEASLES.

MOUNTAIN FEVER. See COLORADO TICK FEVER.

MS. See MULTIPLE SCLEROSIS.

MULTIPLE SCLEROSIS (MS). A chronic, not uncommon disease of the nervous system, multiple sclerosis acts differently in different people, but frequently affects vision, speech, arm and hand movements, and locomotion. It generally hits patients in their thirties, mildly at first, then more severely. The course is irregularly but progressively downhill, but often with periods of marked and prolonged improvement. With some patients partial or complete paralysis is the final outcome; with others a fairly normal life-style is maintained almost indefinitely. When death occurs, it is usually from some secondary cause such as a bacterial infection. Although the matter is not completely settled, it seems likely that a viral infection—possibly by the MEASLES virus—is at least partly responsible, but MS cannot be considered infectious in the usual sense.

Because the disease is so variable, symptoms can begin in any of a number of ways—with slurring of speech, with mistiness or double vision, with numbness or tingling of the muscles, with unsteadiness, dizziness, even vertigo, or with loss of bladder or bowel control. Often, however, such early symptoms clear up completely, and the disease remains in remission for some months or years. But the symptoms generally return, and with increased intensity. Now there may be a pronounced lack of coordination, with tremors, even muscle spasms, and in time paralysis of the affected limbs ensues. Pain of varying intensity may be present, but this is usually not the patient's major complaint.

There is no cure for multiple sclerosis, but treatment can help the patient minimize his disability. Many different drugs have been employed in this disease, but it is difficult to judge their effectiveness because the course of the disease is so variable. Steroids, namely cortisone and related compounds, are often used to reduce the intensity of acute attacks, but prolonged use of steroids brings serious side effects and demands careful supervision. A diet low in saturated fats and high in unsaturated ones has been said to be helpful. Whereas avoidance of fatigue and stress are urged, the patient may be given a program of mild exercise.

The observed symptoms result from attacks on the central nervous system, particularly the nerve fibers in the brain and spinal cord. The outer covering of such fibers, the so-called myelin sheath, is attacked and the fiber itself exposed. Hard (sclerotic) patches appear on the fibers at the multiple points of attack. The particular sites that happen to be attacked dictate the symptoms produced.

There is some indication that this attack is an action of the body's immunity system misdirected against some of its own components; hence MS is sometimes classed as an "autoimmune" disorder. Although no one knows for sure, it is suspected that the autoimmune response is triggered off by a virus infection of the nervous system. Possibly the virus alters the surface of the nerve cells so that the immune system no longer recognizes them as a normal body component, and mounts its attack.

Supporting the theory of virus responsibility are the observations that most multiple sclerosis patients have had previous measles attacks, and the finding of high levels of *antibodies* to the measles virus in many MS patients. In fact, the measles virus itself has been found in the intestines of some such patients. Taken together, this evidence would suggest that MS is a kind of SLOW VIRUS DISEASE caused by the measles virus long after its initial assault on the body.

Unfortunately, this picture is somewhat clouded by the fact that MS patients generally show high levels of antibodies to many common viruses, not just the measles virus. And some investigators have evidence that a second, so far rather mysterious, virus may be involved instead of, or along with, the measles virus. Consistent with this hypothesis is a recent report that an unexpectedly large percentage of MS victims have been closely exposed to a household pet some months before the initial attack. This report would seem to implicate an animal virus in the disease.

Exactly why multiple sclerosis develops in some persons and not others, especially if it is caused by a common virus like the measles virus, is not known. Actually, according to some studies, MS results from a measles infection at a relatively advanced age, and this may be part of the answer. (Interestingly enough, another degenerative nerve disease SUBACUTE SCLEROSING PANENCEPHALITIS seems to result from measles attacks at an unusually early age.) What seems to be involved here mainly, however, is a matter of inherited susceptibility— not that the disease itself is hereditary, but that an abnormality of the immunity or the nervous system is, and that this makes it possible for the virus (or viruses) to produce the disorder in affected individuals.

MUMPS (INFECTIOUS PAROTITIS). An acute, contagious virus disease, mild and of short duration, mumps is notable because it causes swelling of the salivary glands, especially the parotid glands, which are located at the upper corner of the jaw, just below the ear. In children the swelling is somewhat painful and likely to make swallowing difficult, but the disease usually passes quickly and causes no permanent damage. In those beyond the age of puberty, mumps is likely to be more severe and complications are common. Men frequently experience involvement of the testes, and women sometimes undergo swellings of the breasts and ovaries. On rare occasions the pancreas is involved, and EN-CEPHALITIS has been known to occur. Usually these secondary effects are not prolonged, and clear up without aftereffects. The only serious difficulty is that a very few men in whom both testes are affected become impotent or sterile. Fortunately a good vaccine is available, and there is no reason why all susceptible adolescent boys and young men should not be protected. Nonetheless, there is some indication that the vaccine is not being used as widely as it should.

One attack of the disease gives lifelong immunity, whether or not both parotid glands are involved. Hence there is no substance to the old wives' tale that those infected in only one parotid can have the disease again "on the other side." The disease, in fact, is bodywide, not just a local infection of the parotid glands. Some cases show no inflammation of the parotids, and many are completely *inapparent,* though these individuals too are fully protected.

Mumps was known to the ancient Greeks. A very clear clinical description is given by Hippocrates, including an account of testicular involvement.

Generally, the symptoms come on quickly, after an *incubation period* of some 16 to 18 days. The first symptoms often are fever, headache, and a general sense of discomfort. The patient may have a dry cough at this stage and believe he is coming down with a cold. The first indication of parotid involvement is likely to be an earache, but soon the swelling itself becomes obvious as the gland balloons, pushing the ear upward and outward. Then the swelling moves down the side of the jaw as other salivary glands become inflamed. The more pronounced the swelling, the greater the pain—in any case, the swollen area is likely to be tender and sore to the touch; chewing and swallowing usually are painful. There is no discharge, either externally or through the parotid ducts inside the cheek. In most cases the glands at both sides of the jaw are involved; often, however, one is more grossly enlarged than the other.

The disease seldom persists beyond 10 days, and the fever, which is usually not excessive, often subsides before the swelling does. When complications appear, they may come before, with, or after the swelling of the parotids; sometimes they even occur when those glands are not affected.

Inflammation of the testes is the most common complication. It occurs in about 20 percent of infected mature males, but in only about one tenth of these are both testes involved. The infected gland swells rapidly, often to four times its normal size, and becomes painful and tender. The pain and swelling disappear in four or five days, but the tenderness may remain for some time. In about half the patients, the gland ultimately resumes its normal size and function, but in the remainder it largely withers away. This does not seriously affect function, however, unless both glands are so affected, an extremely rare occurrence.

In women, slight breast swelling and tenderness indicate involvement of that gland, and lower abdominal pain, nausea, and vomiting result from ovarial inflammation. When it is the right ovary that is infected, the result may resemble appendicitis. Such localized swellings almost invariably create no major problems and disappear quickly.

When the virus invades the central nervous system, which it does in about 10 percent of all cases, symptoms of encephalitis result. Muscular pain and weakness and even transient paralysis may be observed. Some mental confusion may result also; convulsions are rare. Although most patients recover rapidly and completely, the fatality rate from mumps encephalitis is 1 percent, and a few patients show continued muscular weakness or permanent personality changes. When the pancreas is attacked, abdominal pain and tenderness are found, and the patient often experiences repeated waves of vomiting. Such effects do not continue for long, however, and the patient almost invariably recovers within a week.

The presence of *antibodies* to the mumps virus in individuals not known to have had the disease testifies to the prevalence of inapparent infections. This has been confirmed in children who have been deliberately exposed to forestall the more serious complications faced by adults. After the normal incubation period, the virus could be isolated from about 40 percent of such patients even though they showed none of the usual symptoms. The rest, of course, underwent the typical clinical infection.

Man is the only host of the mumps virus; no animals harboring it have ever been found. The disease is *endemic* in most of the world, with major outbreaks occurring in different localities at intervals of seven or eight years. The disease does not appear to be as common as certain others—measles, for example—but this is probably due to the large numbers of inapparent infections, since most adults tested have antibodies to the virus. The disease is capable of hitting people of any age—recorded ages of victims range from 1 day to 99 years; but it is commonly a disease of the 5- to 10-year-old. Infants are rarely attacked, possibly being protected by maternal antibodies, and the older members of the population usually have already been exposed. The disease seems to favor the winter and spring, though cases can occur at any time.

The saliva is heavily laden with viruses, especially in the few days preceding the appearance of symptoms, and the virus is spread via saliva droplets emitted into the air or by direct contact with saliva or saliva contaminated objects. Although the disease is not highly communicable, the many people with inapparent infections are often infective, and in most cases the viruses are shed before the infection itself is noticed. Most *epidemics* are maintained by schoolchildren. Students in boarding schools and other institutions are especially vulnerable. Young military recruits are often infected at camps.

The role of the virus in causing the symptoms is typical. The virus particles enter through the nose and throat, multiply in the local mucous membranes and lymphatics, produce a *viremia*, and then concentrate on certain target organs, in this case the parotid glands, the gonads, the pancreas, and the tissues of the central nervous system. It has been suggested that infection of the parotids is a local occurrence resulting from direct invasion through the parotid duct in the cheek, but this seems unlikely because of the long incubation period, the joint appearance of parotid swelling and the symptoms of viremia (headache and fever), and the sometimes simultaneous invasion of such distant organs as the testes.

Both *killed-* and *live-virus vaccines* are available. The former must be given as three separate injections, and protection does not persist. Better are the single-dose live vaccines, which are in use in the United States and the Soviet Union. The United State vaccine, which was introduced in 1968, produces protective antibodies in 98 percent of those vaccinated, causes no detectable illness, and gives protection for at least a year or two. It is not yet clear how long immunity produced by this vaccine lasts, but if booster injections are given every few years, it may be for some time.

Up to now, it has often been argued that it is better for young children to experience the disease itself, since it is mild and confers lifelong immunity, rather than be vaccinated and receive only limited protection, thereby possibly postponing the disease to a time when serious complications are more likely. Possibly for these reasons, the best estimates are that only about 35 percent of children in the United States are vaccinated.

Yet it is clear that the only real chance of eradicating the disease completely is through extensive vaccination—and since there is no animal host, this is a feasible goal. As for subsequent risk to those vaccinated, booster injections would certainly restore waning immunity, and at any rate, infections in those once vaccinated are likely to be mild and devoid of complications. So mumps vaccination programs should be vigorously pursued.

There is no specific therapy for mumps. Aspirin and codeine reduce the pain of the parotitis, and warm or cool applications also help. Special treatment may be called for in cases with severe complication. Intravenous feeding may be resorted to, for example, if prolonged vomiting is caused by pancreatitis. *Immune globulin* drawn from convalescent mumps patients is given routinely to infected adult males and occasionally to others to reduce the possibility of complications.

Usually the parotitis itself is enough to ensure correct diagnosis of the disease, especially when an epidemic is in progress. But other diseases, such as adenitis, resemble mumps; and, of course, some patients never develop the parotid swelling. Therefore, there is some reason for undertaking laboratory diagnosis, which can be conclusive. The usual procedures are virus isolation and, more commonly, *serologic tests* for antibodies to the virus. A characteristic skin reaction generally occurs when persons who have previously had the disease are injected with inactivated virus. This reaction is not useful in diagnosis, but it does identify individuals who are immune as a result of previous infection.

The virus—of which there is only one known type—can be cultivated in *tissue culture* or in chicken eggs. It appears to be a typical *RNA* virus of the myxovirus group, much resembling the parainfluenza viruses (see RESPIRATORY INFECTION). The variable diameter of the virus particle, including *outer envelope,* which is covered with small projections, ranges from 100 to 250 nanometers (four to ten millionths of an inch). The inner *helical* coil of protein and RNA has a diameter of about 16 nanometers.

MURRAY VALLEY ENCEPHALITIS. See ST. LOUIS EN-CEPHALITIS.

MYALGIA, EPIDEMIC. See PLEURODYNIA.

MYOCARDITIS. See COXSACKIE OR ECHO VIRUS INFECTION, HEART DISEASE.

NEWCASTLE DISEASE. A highly contagious, but relatively mild, disorder that mainly affects chickens and other poultry, Newcastle disease is occasionally spread to man. In human beings it produces an inflammation of the membranes of the eye (conjunctivitis), or a slight, influenzalike respiratory disease (see RESPIRATORY INFECTION).

Named for Newcastle upon Tyne, England, the site of an early outbreak among chicken flocks, Newcastle disease in chickens causes a disorder with respiratory distress—coughing, sneezing, gasping—as well as nervous system impairment—staggering, stupor, possibly paralysis. Death rates in chickens average only about 5 percent, but because the disease is so widespread, this can mean an appreciable loss of birds. Also, egg-laying is reduced or stopped in sick birds.

The virus is spread via droplets emitted into the air. Veterinary vaccines are available, but the disease is so rare and so mild in man that human-use vaccines have not been developed.

OMSK HEMORRHAGIC FEVER. See HEMORRHAGIC FEVER.

O'NYONG-NYONG VIRUS INFECTION. See DENGUE.

ORF. See PUSTULAR DERMATITIS.

OSTEITIS DEFORMANS. See PAGET'S DISEASE OF BONE.

OSTEOARTHRITIS. See ARTHRITIS.

PAGET'S DISEASE OF BONE (OSTEITIS DEFORMANS). A severe crippling disorder, Paget's disease of bone—there is another Paget's disease, a precancerous condition of the nipple of the breast—is progressive but rarely fatal. Its cause has long been a mystery, but there is now evidence that the disease is due to a virus, possibly the MEASLES virus.

Named for its discoverer, Sir James Paget, a British surgeon, Paget's disease begins in the bone marrow and soon extends into the bones themselves. It causes a simultaneous thinning out and extension of the bone substance, with the result that long, weight-bearing bones become weakened and bowed. Particularly affected are the leg bones, which—in extreme cases—reach up to twice their normal length, though they are badly bent, and the skull bones, which become progressively enlarged.

The disease, which strikes typically between the ages of 40 and 60, affects 3 percent of the population past the age of 40. The ultimate effect is a severe crippling and marked deformity (the medical name, osteitis deformans, means "deforming inflammation of the bones"), and there is often pain in the bones. Other than headache, however, the patient may experience no signs of ill health. Fractures of the weakened bones are not uncommon, and the fatalities that occur are generally from secondary anemia or bone cancer.

That a virus may be involved in the disease is indicated by the repeated findings in the electron microscope of viruslike material in the nuclei of certain bone cells of patients with Paget's disease but not of those with other bone diseases. This material, which is composed of rodlike particles that look exactly like the inner core of the measles virus, much resembles material observed in the nuclei of nerve cells of patients suffering from SUBACUTE SCLEROSING PANENCEPHALITIS. There is other evidence suggesting that this latter disease is caused by the measles virus. By analogy, then, Paget's disease of bone is thought to be also due to the measles virus, or some other virus that much resembles it.

PAPILLOMAS. See WARTS.

PARAINFLUENZA VIRUS INFECTION. See RESPIRATORY INFECTION.

PARALYSIS AGITANS. See PARKINSON'S DISEASE.

PARKINSON'S DISEASE (PARKINSONISM, PARALYSIS AGITANS, SHAKING PALSY). A rather common degenerative disorder of the nervous system, Parkinson's disease is marked by a combination of symptoms that is unmistakable: a slow, shuffling gait; constant tremor of the hands and feet; a slight back-and-forth movement of the head; a stooping posture, with the arms carried in front of the body; and a fixed, blank, unblinking expression. The disease hits about one person in a thousand, with most victims between the ages of 50 and 70. Although a virus cause is suspected, this has not been proved. Recently, great success has been achieved in treating Parkinson's disease with a substance called levodopa, or L-Dopa. This material does not cure Parkinsonism, but it does correct the symptoms to a large extent, and it permits many patients to lead relatively normal lives.

Parkinsonism begins rather slowly with a slight tremor in the hand or a minor dragging of a foot. This may occur as early as age 30, but it generally comes much later. Over the next 10 or 20 years, the condition worsens, with manual dexterity and locomotion affected first—the handwriting becomes small, the gait slows markedly. In time, the patient finds it difficult to rise from a chair or from bed, and experiences frequent falls due to loss of balance. He may sit in the same position for long periods staring straight ahead, but his mind is not affected, and he remains intelligent and alert. His life span may not be appreciably shortened by the disease, and death is almost sure to come from some other cause.

This strange malady was first described in the early nineteenth century by a British general practitioner, James Parkinson, who called it "shaking palsy," or more formally "paralysis agitans." The disease remained relatively rare for about a hundred years, until 1916, when an epidemic of viral ENCEPHALITIS lethargica broke out and left large numbers of people with Parkinson's disease as a delayed aftereffect. Although encephalitis lethargica, and presumably the virus that caused it, disappeared from the scene around 1930, cases of Parkinsonism have continued to appear. According to some studies, the new cases occur in increasingly older age groups, suggesting that they all may arise from exposure to the encephalitis lethargica virus in the years before 1930. (Conceivably, even those with no history of having had that disease could have been exposed to the virus and later develop Parkinsonism.) If this hypothesis is correct, and the matter is far from settled, and if the putative virus has indeed vanished, then Parkinsonism too should very soon disappear.

Most authorities feel, however, that whereas the encephalitis lethargica virus may have been responsible for a bulge of cases of Parkinsonism in the years shortly after it was active, most instances of the disease today stem from some other cause, possibly an as yet unidentified virus. Largely by analogy with other degenerative nervous system diseases, Parkinson's disease is now commonly classed as a SLOW VIRUS DISEASE.

The development of levodopa as a drug for treating Parkinsonism is itself an interesting story. It began when investigators discovered that Parkinson's disease patients uniformly had a deficit of a substance called dopamine, an essential transmitter of nerve impulses, in the brain, and sought ways of correcting that fault. Dopamine itself could not be administered directly to patients because it would not move from the bloodstream into the brain. But after much research it was discovered that the closely related material levodopa would do so and, in fact, in the brain would be converted to dopamine, making up the deficit.

Introduction of levodopa on a large scale in 1970 caused a virtual revolution in the treatment of Parkinsonism. Up to 60 percent of those receiving the drug achieve noticeable relief from their symptoms, and many find themselves able to resume activities they have been unable to carry out for years. Nonetheless, there are drawbacks. Few patients experience full remission of the Parkinson symptoms, and use of the drug is limited in some patients because they develop side effects.

PAROTITIS, INFECTIOUS. See MUMPS.

PERICARDITIS. See COXSACKIE OR ECHO VIRUS INFECTION, HEART DISEASE.

PHLEBOTOMUS FEVER. See SANDFLY FEVER.

PLEURODYNIA (EPIDEMIC MYALGIA, BORNHOLM DISEASE, DEVIL'S GRIP). Pleurodynia is an infectious disease characterized by fever, headache, nausea, cough, and stabbing chest pain. It hits all age groups, but is especially prevalent among children and young adults. Symptoms generally last only about a week, and recovery is rapid and complete. The disease is caused by certain coxsackie viruses (see COXSACKIE OR ECHO VIRUS INFECTION).

Although pleurodynia was reported as early as the 18th century, the first epidemic to be fully described occurred on the Danish island of Bornholm in 1930. Since then, epidemics have been reported in many parts of the world, but the disease is not common.

A few patients experience fever, headache, and a general sense of illness before the chest pain appears—the literal meaning of "pleurodynia" is chest pain—but for most people the sudden attack of pain is the first sign of illness. It is variously described as "a stitch in the side" or "like being squeezed in a tight grip." General muscular aches (myalgia) almost always occur, and sometimes the sharp pain is chiefly abdominal. Sore throat, cough, even hiccoughs, may be present. A moderate fever usually persists for as long as the pain is present— anywhere from two days to two weeks. Vomiting and nausea are rare. Some patients experience stiffness of the back and neck, and other signs of MENINGITIS. In males, pain and tenderness of the testes is an occasional complication. Invariably, symptoms pass with time, and recovery is complete. There is no special treatment for the disease, though aspirin and other pain-killing drugs may be used when needed.

Sporadic epidemics of pleurodynia have been observed in Europe,

North America, and Australia, chiefly in the summer months. Nearly all the so-called coxsackie B viruses, six of which are known, have been associated with outbreaks of the disease, and it has been reported that on rare occasion coxsackie A viruses have been involved. Probably the causative viruses multiply in the muscles of the chest wall, producing the characteristic symptoms of the disease. As in the case of other coxsackie virus infections, transmission is presumed to be by way of the stools, though emission of viruses from the throat by coughing cannot be ruled out. The virus most likely enters the body through the mouth or the upper respiratory tract.

The chest pain alone is often enough to identify the disease, but when there is abdominal pain, confusion with appendicitis can result, especially since pleurodynia may be accompanied by a rigidity of the abdominal muscles, another sign of appendicitis. In the laboratory, the presence of coxsackie viruses can be confirmed by injection of material from stools into newborn mice, who develop characteristic abnormalities in response. Also, *serologic tests* show a rise of *antibodies* to coxsackie viruses during the course of the ailment. Since any of the six coxsackie B viruses seem able to cause pleurodynia, a successful vaccine would have to protect against all of them—and so far, no such vaccine has been developed.

PML. See PROGRESSIVE MULTIFOCAL LEUKOENCE-PHALOPATHY.

PNEUMONIA. See RESPIRATORY INFECTION.

POLIO (POLIOMYELITIS, INFANTILE PARALYSIS). An acute infectious disease of children and young adults, polio is a disorder of remarkable variability. Most people who have it notice no symptoms at all; some experience a disease like THE COMMON COLD or INFLUENZA; and a few are subject to temporary or permanent paralysis. The death rate is very low.

In the early decades of the 20th century, great *epidemics* of polio swept the cities of North America and Europe each summer, leaving thousands of paralyzed victims. Then, in the 1950s and early 1960s, development of the Salk and Sabin vaccines brought such epidemics under control—but the disease remains *endemic* in many parts of the world. Constant maintenance of vaccination programs is still necessary, however, to prevent resurgence of the disease in epidemic form.

There is little doubt that polio is very old; it has probably existed in much of the world for millennia. A stone carving from ancient Egypt shows a man with a withered leg exactly like that of some modern polio sufferer.

The disease was first described by Michael Underwood, a British physician, in 1789 and, more completely, by Jakob von Heine, a German orthopedist, in 1840. That polio was infectious was first recognized in 1890 by a Swedish physician, Oscar Medin, who reported on an epidemic in Stockholm. (For a time polio was known as the Heine-Medin disease.) It is possible that the Stockholm epidemic observed by Medin was the first major polio epidemic to have occurred, the disease up to that time having existed only in endemic form.

In 1909 Karl Landsteiner and Erwin Popper in Vienna succeeded in transmitting polio to monkeys, and that same year Landsteiner and Constantin Levaditi showed that the disease is caused by a virus. In 1949 John Franklin Enders and two associates at Harvard University Medical School discovered how to grow the virus in *tissue culture*, a feat that won for them the 1954 Nobel Prize in Medicine and paved the way for development of polio vaccines.

The first vaccine, a *killed-virus vaccine* prepared by Jonas Salk, was tested in the United States on a large scale in 1954; and the following year, with much ballyhoo from the National Foundation for Infantile Paralysis, which had supported Salk's work with its annual March of Dimes fund-raising events, the vaccine was launched in a nationwide campaign. Having "Salk shots" was now required of all schoolchildren. Regrettably, the early days of the campaign were marred by several hundred cases of polio and eleven deaths caused by the vaccine. Unforseen complication in the scaling up of Salk's procedure and inadequate testing had led to live viruses in the supposedly inactivated vaccine.

Yet, on the whole, the Salk vaccine worked well. The manufacturing problems proved not to be insoluble, and with proper safeguards, mass vaccinations continued for several years in the United States and many other countries. In the United States alone 79,000 people were paralyzed from polio in the five years before introduction of the Salk vaccine; in the next five years, only 21,000 were, a reduction of 75 percent. In Sweden, polio was virtually eliminated by the Salk vaccine.

But there are inherent drawbacks to the Salk vaccine. To begin with, it is given by injection—two or three separate shots, a month apart, followed by a "booster" six months later. (To maintain protection, repeated booster injections may be needed.) This is inconvenient in any mass immunization program and all but impossible in an underdeveloped country.

Further, the Salk vaccine produces immunity in the blood but not in the intestinal tract, where the virus multiplies. *Wild* polio *viruses* are thus able to invade the bodies of vaccinees, multiply in the gut, and pass out in the stools, possibly infecting new victims. In the original vaccinees, the blood immunity produced by the vaccine blocks access to the nervous system by wild viruses, thereby preventing paralytic symptoms. But in those exposed to wild viruses from the vaccinees, no such protection exists, and paralytic polio may result. In short, the Salk vaccine protects the vaccinated, but fails to stop them from spreading the disease to others.

In the late 1950s, while the Salk vaccine was being introduced, Albert Sabin—then at the University of Cincinnati's College of Medicine—was at work on an oral *live-virus vaccine*, which he hoped would overcome the disadvantages of the Salk vaccine. (Actually, Sabin's was not the first live polio vaccine; one had been developed by Hilary Koprowski at Lederle Laboratories in 1950, but the Sabin vaccine proved to be superior.) Large-scale testing of the Sabin vaccine was carried out in 1960 in the United States, and the vaccine was widely used in Russia, beginning in that year. In 1962 it was licensed for use in the United States, and it soon came to be employed virtually everywhere in the world to the almost total exclusion of the Salk vaccine.

Administered on sugar lumps, as drops, or in capsules, the Sabin vaccine is easy to handle in large programs. Also, because the vaccine consists of live (but weakened) viruses, which themselves multiply in the gut, it produces localized intestinal immunity and therefore prevents the subsequent growth of wild, disease-producing polio viruses there. Thus, those vaccinated with Sabin vaccine, unlike Salk vaccinees, are not only immune to paralytic polio themselves; they also serve as barriers to spread of the virus. In fact, the Sabin vaccine causes immunity to develop so quickly (usually within a week, much more quickly than the Salk vaccine) that it is capable of halting epidemics that are just beginning.

As is true of any vaccine, the Sabin vaccine cannot be considered 100 percent safe. A very few cases of polio—even paralytic polio—have developed in vaccinees, but the rate is very low. Because the polio virus exists in three forms, or types, full protection can be assured only when the individual is vaccinated against all three. Originally the Sabin procedure called for the three types to be given as separate doses of so-called monovalent vaccine, but when this was done, it was found that the type-3 vaccine caused some trouble. (With the type-3 vaccine, the paralytic polio rate in vaccinees was slightly higher—one in a million.) It has now been found safer to give the three types together in a trivalent vaccine (as is done with the Salk vaccine). In the trivalent form the type-3 strain is less likely to cause difficulty, presumably because the other strains prevent the type-3 virus from initiating a full-scale infection. (The trivalent vaccine also, of course, offers considerable logistical advantage in mass vaccination campaigns: stock of three separate vaccines need no longer be differentiated, and complex vaccination schedules need not be adhered to.) All in all, the Sabin vaccine is, as one authority puts it, "one of the safer immunologic preparations available."

Typically, the trivalent vaccine is given according to the following schedule: beginning at the age of about three months (at earlier ages the infant carries maternal *antibodies* that would inactivate any live vaccine), the child receives two or three doses of vaccine six to eight weeks apart. Then, about a year later, a third or fourth dose is given. And, finally, when the child is ready to start school, he gets a final "booster" dose. This course has been established as safe and productive of high levels of immunity.

There might seem to be little basis for arguing with the success of the Sabin vaccine. In the United States, for example, introduction of the Salk vaccine brought the average annual number of paralytic cases down from about 15,000 to about 4,000; then, in 1961 when the Sabin vaccine began to be used to head off budding epidemics, the number of paralytic cases fell below 1,000 for the first time. Mass vaccination campaigns then followed, in which 100 million Americans received the Sabin vaccine in a year and a half, and the number of cases fell below 100—almost all being unvaccinated individuals—a level at which it has remained, in spite of some slackening of the vaccination level. (Public health officials in the United States warn, however, that the pace of vaccinations is not high enough to maintain protection in the face of possible new epidemics.) Similar successes have been achieved wherever the Sabin vaccine has come into general use.

Yet recently, Jonas Salk has launched a campaign against the Sabin vaccine, charging that it is unsafe. The odds against acquiring paralytic polio from the vaccine, however, are very small, one in 11.5 million, according to one estimate. Furthermore, most authorities are convinced that the Salk vaccine, even if it should prove safer, could not do as good a job as the Sabin vaccine has done in protecting the United States against polio.

Most infections by the polio virus go unrecognized—it is estimated that 90 to 95 percent of polio infections are *inapparent*—i.e., symptomless. Evidence that this is the case arises when mass screening programs detect antibodies to the virus in the blood of persons who have never been infected or vaccinated. When symptoms do appear, they are likely to be only cold- or flu-like and to persist for a few hours or days. This so-called "minor illness" of polio is characterized by various combinations of fever, headache, nausea, vomiting, sore throat, constipation, and muscle pains. When these constitute the only symptoms, the disease is again likely to go undiagnosed—unless a polio epidemic is in progress or unless laboratory tests for the virus are run.

Even more serious cases of polio are likely to begin with the minor illness, which subsides as usual and is then followed by a three- or four-day interval without apparent signs. Then, however, the early symptoms return, in aggravated form—higher fever, more severe headache, and so on. This so-called "major illness," which sometimes appears at once, without the minor phase, is usually accompanied by ENCEPHALITIS, inflammation of the brain, or—more commonly—by MENINGITIS, irritation of the membranes surrounding the brain and spinal cord. Signs of encephalitis include headache, drowsiness, behavioral changes; of meningitis, stiffness and pain in the back and neck. This phase of the disease may persist for four or five days, and then pass without further symptoms. Or, in the case of some 1 percent of the overall number infected, it is the prelude to temporary or permanent paralysis.

Although paralysis is generally a late symptom, it may appear at any time within the first week of major illness. It is rarely the first sign (though this has occurred), being usually preceded at least by fever and stiffness of the back and neck. If the period of major illness passes without paralysis, as occurs in about one case in four, the patient is assured that that symptom will not appear. Acute muscle pain is often present, however, and, by affecting the patient's will to move the affected muscles, may mask the paralysis.

Paralysis generally develops quickly, reaching its maximum in three days. With cessation of the fever, a slow recovery of function begins, usually reaching a plateau in about six months, though improvement may continue for as long as two years.

The nature of the paralysis varies from case to case. Most commonly affected are the nerves that govern the muscles of the upper parts of the legs; next most commonly affected, the nerves of the muscles of the upper arms and shoulders. After this come attacks on the nerves of the chest muscles, whose failure may lead to a stop in breathing. Least common are attacks on (1) the facial nerves, (2) the nerves that control swallowing and speaking, and (3) the nerves that directly maintain breathing and the heartbeat.

The extent and duration of paralysis also vary. Paralysis that affects the heart or breathing mechanism is most serious, and it is in such cases that most fatalities occur. (The number dying is about 5 percent of those who suffer the major illness.) Yet, attacks of this kind often are not so severe, and the patient who survives is likely to recover completely. When the chest muscles are paralyzed and the breath is maintained artificially, some improvement is usually noted for a time, but this may never be great enough to permit unaided respiration. Attacks on limbs are not life threatening, but are most likely to lead to permanent paralysis. The attack is usually on only one side of the body, and the muscles of the affected limb atrophy, leaving the limb shorter and less well developed than its opposite number. In all, some 14 percent of those experiencing the major illness are left with some permanent, incapacitating paralysis.

Several factors have been found to increase the likelihood and severity of paralysis in polio patients, the most important being excessive exercise or other fatiguing activity during the early phase of the major illness. Tonsillectomy, adenoidectomy, and tooth extraction may stimulate paralysis in the nearby muscles, and vaccination or other injections may lead to paralysis in the limb involved. Rest is, therefore, an obvious part of the treatment of those suspected of having polio, and the medical procedures mentioned are best postponed, if possible, in unprotected individuals, when polio appears to be at large.

Treatment of polio, of course, depends on the severity of the attack. Patients experiencing the minor illness need no special care, but for those undergoing the major illness, complete bed rest is a must. The physician will decide if the patient is to be hospitalized—transporting the patient may exhaust him, with serious consequences; but should danger to breathing or the heart arise, hospital facilities may be needed quickly. It is important that a physician's advice be sought when a patient, especially a child, experiences, in the summer months, a cold- or flu-like ailment with stiffness of the back and neck.

Beyond complete rest, there is no special treatment for nonparalytic polio. *Gamma globulin* and *immune serum* are no help once symptoms have appeared. Mild sedatives or tranquilizers may be prescribed to facilitate rest, but they are to be avoided in certain forms of paralytic polio, and the choice must be left to the physician.

Special treatment obviously is called for when paralysis does appear. With paralysis of the limbs, a firm, hard bed is recommended during the phase of feverish illness, and attention should be given to proper positioning of the affected limbs. Care by professional orthopedists and physical therapists is essential during this phase of the disease and the first months of convalescence to assure maximum recovery of disabled muscles. The general methods of treatment employed are (1) application of moist, hot packs over the affected areas and (2) gentle, passive movement of the limbs involved. Above all, rigid immobilization of muscles is to be avoided during this early period. Ultimately, when the maximum amount of muscle use has been regained, braces and splints may be employed for support, and surgery may be resorted to, to equalize disproportionately sized limbs.

Paralysis of the chest muscles may necessitate immediate use of a mechanical respirator during the acute phase, and depending on the degree of recovery, such usage may have to be continued indefinitely. The "iron lung" respirator was an all-too-frequent sign of the polio epidemics of the 1930s and 1940s, and the horror it induced was much exploited by the National Foundation in its fund-raising drives. This large "tank" respirator can often be replaced by a smaller chest respirator, which is less fearsome to the patient. When paralysis occurs in the throat, swallowing becomes impossible and secretions may have to be removed with a suction device to permit the patient to breathe. In extreme cases, tracheotomy may be necessary, and when breathing is also affected, oxygen may have to be administered through the tracheotomy tube.

The behavior of the polio virus in the body and the way it causes the various symptoms are fairly well known. The virus probably enters through the mouth—on food, fingers, or utensils—or, less likely, it is inhaled on droplets in the air. It may multiply to some extent in the throat, but the chief site of multiplication is thought to be the intestinal wall. Up to this stage the action of the virus may lead to no noticeable symptoms at all.

From the intestines, however, the virus may invade the lymph glands and the bloodstream, and a proliferation of the virus in the blood (*viremia*) probably corresponds to the phase of minor illness. Finally, the virus enters the central nervous system, either from the bloodstream directly or possibly from the intestinal tract via nerve pathways. A period of virus multiplication in the tissues of the nervous system seems to correspond with the second phase of the disease, the major illness. The observed signs of encephalitis and meningitis result from direct attack of the virus on the brain or the membrane surrounding it. Paralysis comes from virus damage to specific motor nerve connections in the spinal cord or the brain stem. When the attack is on the lower part of the spinal cord, the limb muscles are affected; when it is on the upper part, the chest muscles. Damage to the brain stem, or "bulb," causes paralysis of the muscles of the face or throat or the centers that regulate the breath and heartbeat. (Often polio is classed as "spinal" or "bulbar" depending on which of these two patterns is observed.) The amount of viral damage to nerve cells dictates the extent and severity of the paralysis.

Epidemiologically—that is, in its patterns of spread—polio behaves almost like two separate diseases. On the one hand, we have the highly visible, epidemic disease of North America and Europe, with its yearly outbreaks in the summer months; on the other, the endemic, year-round but little regarded disease of the underdeveloped countries. The difference is largely caused by variations in sanitary practice, but it may also reflect two different modes of transmission.

It has been amply demonstrated that, because of the intestinal nature of the infection, viruses are discharged in the stools for several weeks whether or not symptoms appear. When sanitation is poor, and families are large and overcrowded, the virus undoubtedly spreads by fecal contamination of bodies, foodstuffs, water, utensils, and the living quarters themselves. (Flies may help move the virus around the living area, too.) Under such circumstances the virus is very easily taken in by mouth, and almost every child is exposed at an early age. In fact, many children may be first exposed while still protected by maternal antibodies; they then experience mild infections, which stimulate production of their own antibodies and offer protection against later attacks. Serious illnesses, paralysis, and even deaths undoubtedly do occur, but they are scattered among a very large population, most of whom experience no illness from the disease at all, and polio as a separate entity is hardly observed among the myriad of childhood diseases.

When sanitation is good and personal cleanliness an easy-to-indulge habit, rapid spread of the virus by the fecal-oral route is inhibited. Viruses may fail to circulate for a considerable period of time, until a large crop of susceptible individuals has built up. Then the virus appears afresh, probably from some area where it is endemic, and finds waiting for it a fertile new home. Here, too, the virus may spread by the fecal-oral route—children are the main spreaders of virus in any polio epidemic—or it may move by the second route: droplet emission from the nose and throat. It is known that the virus is present in the upper respiratory area for a few days early in the infection, and it is possible—experts are divided on this point—that enough viruses are emitted during coughing and sneezing to contaminate the air space. At any rate, under this set of conditions, the virus now is capable of truly explosive growth—it encounters a great many susceptible individuals and moves among them like a chain reaction.

Apparently, until the late 19th century, conditions were not right for the epidemic pattern of polio to appear. Then, with the development of the first large cities with modern sanitation, the great polio epidemics began, first in Stockholm, as noted, then in comparable cities around the world. Now, as health care and sanitary conditions improve everywhere, new countries, one by one, find themselves moving from regions of endemic polio to ones where polio epidemics prevail.

The reason that epidemics occur chiefly in the summer months, whereas the endemic disease is found year-round, is probably climate. The summer epidemic pattern exists largely in the temperate zones, but the year-round endemic pattern is chiefly tropical. Apparently the virus is less easily transmitted, or more easily inactivated, during cold weather.

Considering the large areas where polio is endemic—the virus has been found in every country in which it has been sought—the possibility of completely eliminating the disease soon is not great. Yet the Sabin vaccine offers hope that this might someday be accomplished. Oral vaccination does produce immune persons who act as barriers to the spread of the disease, and since there are no known animal hosts in which the virus can maintain itself, worldwide immunization campaigns could ultimately eliminate the virus completely. But a truly massive effort to accomplish this result would be required.

Diagnosing polio is not difficult when the paralytic symptoms are present, as only a few other diseases cause paralysis of the same kind. Now that extensive polio vaccination has drastically reduced the number of cases, however, the other diseases that do cause paralysis are comparatively more common and diagnosis is no longer so simple. It is now recognized that many poliolike attacks are really infections by echo and coxsackie viruses (see COXSACKIE OR ECHO VIRUS INFECTION). Furthermore, several varieties of ARBOVIRUS DISEASE sometimes also produce brief localized paralysis. Finally, there is a somewhat mysterious disorder of uncertain origin, known as the GUILLAIN-BARRÉ SYNDROME, which resembles polio to some extent.

The Guillain-Barré syndrome can be differentiated from polio fairly readily. It is more likely than polio to affect both sides of the body to the same extent; it is usually not accompanied by pain; and it causes characteristic changes in the cerebrospinal fluid. The other causes of paralytic disease, however, are more difficult to distinguish from polio, and reliance is increasingly placed on viral diagnostic procedures.

When the paralytic symptoms are absent, laboratory diagnosis is even more important, especially now that actual polio epidemics are infrequent. (During an epidemic, it is rather easy to infer that a mild case of poliolike disease is, in fact, polio.) Although the signs of meningitis and encephalitis suggest polio, they can also be indications of MUMPS, echo, coxsackie, or arbovirus infection, or any number of other disorders. (Mumps of course is usually, though not invariably, accompanied by a swelling of the jaw, and it is mainly a winter disease.) When encephalitis and meningitis are absent, the remaining symptoms could represent so many diseases that laboratory diagnosis is a necessity.

The most likely place to find polio viruses is in the patient's stools. Throat swabs are sometimes taken, but the chance of picking up viruses is less good; and the blood rarely contains viruses (since the stage of active viremia occurs during the early or minor phase of illness, before polio is likely to be suspected). When encephalitis or meningitis is present, cerebrospinal fluid usually is taken. Characteristic changes in the cell count and the protein levels help differentiate polio from Guillain-Barré syndrome and other diseases, and although polio viruses are rarely found in cerebrospinal fluid, echo or coxsackie viruses frequently are.

The presence of polio viruses in the material from the patient is demonstrated by adding it to cells grown in tissue culture, usually monkey kidney cells, and observing the changes that occur. Positive identification of the virus is given by showing that its activity is blocked by antibodies to one of the known types of polio virus.

Another way of diagnosing polio in the laboratory is by way of *serologic tests* that reveal a sharp rise in antibodies to one of the known virus types during the course of the infection. For this purpose, blood samples are drawn and tested early and late in the infection.

Although the polio virus infects only man in nature, other animals can be infected in the laboratory. At first only monkeys and chimpanzees could be so infected, but now virus strains have been adapted to mice and other laboratory animals. Once tissue-culture methods had been developed for growing the virus, they were used exclusively for laboratory study or vaccine manufacture, but monkeys are still used to test vaccines.

Monkey kidney cells are employed for manufacture of both the Salk and Sabin vaccines. One of the problems in both cases is to assure that the monkey cells are free of natural monkey viruses, whose effects on human beings could not be predicted. This problem is considerably greater with the Sabin vaccine, since the viruses are not inactivated during preparation. As might be imagined, considerable consternation was caused when it was discovered that some early lots of polio vaccine, were, in fact, contaminated with the monkey virus SV40, which is known to cause tumors in hamsters. Fortunately, careful studies revealed no indication of cases of human cancer traceable to such vaccines. Nonetheless, monkeys whose kidneys are to be used for vaccine preparation are now quarantined for six weeks or more before the kidneys are taken, and kidney cells are carefully examined at every step of the manufacturing process to assure that known monkey viruses are not present.

For preparation of vaccines of both types, cultures of kidney cells are seeded with vaccine viruses, and these are allowed to grow for appropriate periods and then harvested. To make either vaccine, viruses of the three different strains are grown separately, and when trivalent vaccine is to be prepared, these are mixed to give the final product. For the Salk vaccine, of course, virulent virus strains are used; for the Sabin vaccine, strains that have been attenuated so that they do not produce the more damaging effects, especially paralysis. The Salk procedure includes inactivation of the harvested viruses by a 12- to 15-day treatment with formalin (formaldehyde); the Sabin vaccine uses the live viruses directly. Both vaccines are repeatedly tested for safety and potency during the manufacturing process.

The three types of polio virus are quite closely related, but can be differentiated because the body produces slightly different antibodies to them. Each type causes essentially the same disease, but they are rather unevenly distributed around the world. Type 1 causes the bulk of the cases in the United States and western Europe, though type 2 also occurs there; type 3 is more prevalent in the Middle East and eastern Europe.

The virus particles of the three forms look the same under the electron microscope. They are small (about 30 nanometers, or a millionth of an inch, in diameter) and roughly spherical (*icosahedral*). They contain about one quarter single-stranded *RNA* enclosed in a protein shell, with no *outer envelope*. The first animal virus to be crystallized (in 1955), the polio virus has been extensively studied. It is classified as an enterovirus, or intestinal virus, along with the coxsackie and echo viruses, which it closely resembles physically and in biological behavior.

POLIO, FRENCH. See GUILLAIN-BARRÉ SYNDROME.

POLYARTERITIS. See CONNECTIVE TISSUE DISEASE.

POSTTRANSFUSION HEPATITIS (POSTTRANSFUSION JAUNDICE). See HEPATITIS.

PROGRESSIVE MULTIFOCAL LEUKOENCEPHALOPATHY (PML). A rare disorder, which is generally fatal, progressive multifocal leukoencephalopathy is caused by progressive destruction of the white matter of the brain, leading ultimately to coma and paralysis. It occurs only in patients whose immunity system has been damaged by disease (such as Hodgkin's disease) or by immunosuppressive drugs (those used to prevent rejection of transplants).

This disease is of special interest because the nerve cell destruction, which occurs primarily in the outer covering of the nerve fibers, the so-called myelin sheath, seems to be due to the action of a virus. This virus can be seen in infected cells with the aid of the electron microscope, and it can be grown in *tissue culture*. It has been shown to be related to two viruses that cause tumors in animals, SV40 and the polyoma virus.

In some respects, progressive multifocal leukoencephalopathy resembles PARKINSON'S DISEASE and MULTIPLE SCLEROSIS. It may be somewhat representative of the general category of SLOW VIRUS DISEASE.

PUSTULAR DERMATITIS. Chiefly a disease of sheep and goats—in sheep it is often called orf—pustular dermatitis sometimes attacks farmers, shepherds, meat handlers, and veterinarians. The disease takes the form of one or a very few large, pimplelike sores with a central depression or ulcer. In man these occur on the hand, arm, or eyelid; in sheep on the lips, vulva, and cornea. The sores eventually heal by themselves, although they may last up to two months before doing so. The responsible virus is a very large *DNA* virus in the pox family (see SMALLPOX)—up to 300 nanometers (ten millionths of an inch) in its largest dimension.

RABIES (HYDROPHOBIA). Conveyed to man by the bite of a diseased animal, often a dog, rabies is an infection of the central nervous system and the salivary glands. It generally produces agonizing convulsions or paralysis, sometimes both successively, and is almost invariably fatal. Fortunately, the *incubation period* is long and a course of vaccinations, begun at once after infection, is quite uniformly successful. Until very recently this treatment itself was protracted, painful, and risky, but newer vaccines are making it less so.

It is easy to recognize descriptions of rabies in very old Egyptian, Greek, and Latin texts, which refer to docile animals suddenly (and supposedly supernaturally) becoming vicious, biting people near them, and then succumbing to mania, paralysis, and death. The Roman medical writer Celsus made the connection between such animal bites and the subsequent development of hydrophobia in the victims. As a treatment he suggested immediate cauterization of the wounds (an effective, if drastic, method).

Vaccination against rabies was introduced by Louis Pasteur in 1885.

Five years earlier, at the age of 58 and partially paralyzed from a stroke, Pasteur had taken up the study of rabies, hoping to develop a vaccine as he had done earlier with two animal diseases, anthrax and chicken cholera. To make his vaccine, Pasteur used rabies viruses grown in a series of rabbit brains. These had become adapted to and made more virulent for the rabbit but at the same time had been weakened, or attenuated, for the dogs on which Pasteur experimented—and, he hoped, for man. But to weaken the viruses further, Pasteur dried rabbit spinal cords containing them for various periods of time. The course of vaccinations would begin with the preparations that had dried longest and were least potent, and proceed over a 10-day period using progressively stronger ones.

The first test of the vaccine on a human being came on July 6, 1865, when a nine-year-old Alsatian boy, Joseph Meister, who had been viciously bitten by a rabid dog, was brought to Pasteur by his mother. After much indecision Pasteur began the inoculations, which were completed on July 16. The lad remained well and happy and quickly became devoted to his new friend, "Monsieur Pasteur." On October 26 Pasteur appeared before the French Academy of Sciences to report the successful experiment and to announce that he had just begun the treatment of a second bitten boy (who was also to remain free of rabies). An ironic postscript to the story is that in 1940, when the German army occupied Paris, a group of sight-seeing German soldiers visited the crypt of Pasteur, where the aged Joseph Meister was a porter, and demanded that it be opened; Meister, rather than submit Pasteur's body to the indignity, killed himself.

Pasteur's method of vaccination achieved instant success, and was acclaimed in France and around the world. It was the last and greatest triumph of a life of repeated scientific accomplishment. The rabies vaccine was only the second vaccine to be developed for human use (the first since Jenner's SMALLPOX vaccine of 90 years before). Soon an international appeal had raised 2½ million francs to found the Pasteur Institute in Paris, which opened in 1888 and became the world center for preparation and study of the vaccine. (In time branches were established in the French provinces and abroad.)

As a disease rabies is truly horrible. It is agonizing even to watch. After a variable incubation period—generally one to three months, but possibly as short as six days or as long as one year—symptoms begin: headache, lost of appetite, fever, nausea, and sore throat. The most characteristic early symptom is a peculiar sensation, difficult to describe, in the area of the original bite.

Then, increasingly, the patient shows signs of abnormal functioning of the nervous system, including undue sensitivity to pressure on the skin (he may complain of the mere presence of the bedclothes) and overresponse to loud noises and bright lights. Spasms of the muscles of the throat result from attempts to swallow, and these may become so prolonged, so severe, and so painful that they are all but unbearable. Ultimately, merely the sight of water may be enough to trigger the painful paroxysms, a circumstance that accounts for the alternate name hydrophobia (fear of water).

In time, the seizures increase in severity and extend to generalized convulsions, during which the patient may die of respiratory failure. Often there are quiet times between seizures, and the patient may remain rational to the end. If he survives this period, however, he soon becomes paralyzed and is likely to die in a paralytic coma. In rare instances, especially in cases resulting from bat bites, the nervous overexcitement and convulsions are not observed and increasing paralysis is the predominant symptom. Only one or two instances are recorded of persons who have recovered from the disease.

In dogs the disease is often characterized as "furious" or "dumb," depending on whether excitement or paralysis predominates, although both are usually present to some degree. The symptom of hydrophobia is not a characteristic of dog rabies. Other animals experience varying responses to the virus; *inapparent infections* are thought to occur in some species, but so far they have been observed definitely only in the bat.

There is no doubt that the rabies virus causes extensive destruction in the brain and nervous system, and that this is responsible for the behavioral changes characteristic of the disease. The damage to tissue is clearly visible when specimens are examined under the microscope. If the disease has progressed far enough, clumps of viruses—called Negri bodies after their discoverer, an Italian physician—can be observed within the cells in specially stained preparations of brain tissue. These are most abundant in preparations drawn from that part of the brain known as the hippocampus.

The virus almost always enters the body via bites through the skin, being copiously present in the saliva of rabid animals. Sometimes cut, scratched, or abraded skin comes in contact with virus-laden saliva and infection ensues—this may happen to unprotected veterinarians, farm workers, and other animal handlers. The virus on occasion passes through intact mucous membranes, so that being licked on the lips by a rabid animal may be enough to give one the disease. It is said that rabies has been contracted by eating the flesh of infected animals (though cooking should inactivate the virus). Also, it is suspected that virus particles carried in the air of enclosed spaces can spread the contagion. There is good evidence of people having been exposed in this way in caves frequented by rabid bats, and it seems significant that many of the most commonly infected wild animals, such as foxes, themselves live in burrows.

The primary pathway by which the virus travels in the body is the nervous system—it has been demonstrated that infection is halted when nerves are cut—but there may be some local movement in blood and lymph. Part of the reason for the long (and variable) incubation period is the time the virus takes to actually enter the nervous system; it may lie relatively quiescent in muscle tissue for weeks or months before penetrating a nerve. Once in a nerve, however, the virus multiplies quickly and spreads to the spinal cord and brain. The speed with which this is accomplished depends upon the number of viruses present and their proximity to the central nervous system (though this latter point has been disputed). Deep bites on the head and face are most often followed by quickly developing symptoms.

From its chief focus in the central nervous system, the virus moves outward again along the nerve network, occasionally attacking such organs as the kidneys but concentrating on the salivary glands, where it multiplies extensively. The peculiar combination of brain damage and salivary gland infection is what makes it possible for the virus to move from animal to animal. The nervous excitability and biting behavior induced by the brain damage and the plentiful supply of virus particles in the saliva together assure spread of the contagion.

Although people most frequently get the disease from dogs, cats too carry it. Every kind of higher animal is believed to be susceptible, from the mouse to the elephant, and the disease remains *endemic* at low levels in wild animal species in various parts of the world. From time to time it erupts in major *epidemics,* often involving only one or two animal species. These include, in different parts of the world, and roughly in order of decreasing frequency, the fox, the wolf, the skunk, the mongoose, and the bat. Occasionally such animals attack man directly—campers are especially prone to infection. There are well-documented cases in the United States of campers being bitten by skunks. A boy in a western campground was bitten by one that had crawled into his sleeping bag. Also, the importation of exotic animals for zoos and, increasingly, as pets is a source of rabies in man. In 1965, a score of people in an Edinburgh zoo were exposed by a leopard from Nepal. Mostly, however, wild animals infect man indirectly through his pets or farm animals—besides dogs and cats, cattle, horses, and sheep are all susceptible. Vampire bats infect cattle on a large scale in Central and South America, enough to pose a serious economic problem, and even fruit- and insect-eating bats when rabid bite other animals.

The change in behavior of an infected animal is remarkable: an ordinarily friendly pet becomes furious and uncontrollable, viciously biting its owner, or an aloof one becomes unusually affectionate, licking him about the nose and mouth. A shy nocturnal animal may wander into unfamiliar open territory in broad daylight, and a wild, usually unapproachable creature becomes quite bold, runs up to a stranger, and then without warning turns on him violently. (There are reports of surprised dogs, and people, being attacked furiously by infected rabbits.)

It is this kind of behavior that makes rabid animals such a menace to young children (half those bitten in the United States are under 15). The child is charmed by the animal's unexpectedly friendly behavior and stops to play with it, at which point he is caught off guard by its sudden unprovoked attack. Often children (and adults) are bitten when they decide to look after obviously sick animals, such as bats. Proper warnings about approaching sick or peculiarly behaving wild animals—especially overfriendly ones—would do much to halt human exposure to rabies.

Wanderlust plays a big part in rabies epizootics (animal epidemics). Rabid dogs and wolves, particularly, are prone to take off on long, cross-country trips, stopping at random locations along the way to attack new victims and leaving scores of such foci of infection behind them.

Animal rabies is a growing public health problem in most countries of the world in the 1970s. Even isolated countries like Britain, which are rabies-free and manage to remain so by strict quarantine, must remain constantly vigilant. Dogs that have undergone the mandatory six-month quarantine have been known to develop rabies, either because of the variable incubation period or because of accidental infection during quarantine. And it is almost impossible to maintain longer periods over the violent protests of pet owners—in some countries quarantine of only three or four months is required. Smuggling of pets past quarantine officers does occur, and only a few species are covered by quarantine regulations anyway, so rabies outbreaks can occur in spite of these precautions.

In countries where wild animal rabies is not uncommon, and is in fact increasing, such as the United States, Canada, and much of the rest of the world, quarantine is of little point—the disease is already present; the problem is to keep it from spreading. Under such circumstances, extensive dog and cat vaccination is resorted to, to set up a protective buffer between man and infected wildlife. This, of course, is only partly effective because of the frequent direct exposure of man to rabid wild animals.

Wholesale vaccination in the wild has been used as a means of halting epizootics, but this is an expensive and troublesome procedure because of the difficulty in tracking down and capturing animals. (Vaccination of valuable livestock to protect them from bat-borne rabies is quite common.) Usually epidemics are handled by slaughter of large numbers of the most susceptible species, either by hunting or with poisoned bait, the aim being to reduce the population to a level below what would maintain the epidemic but high enough to permit repopulation of the area when the rabies threat has receded. This procedure is frequently resorted to in Europe to halt epidemics of fox rabies. It seems inhumane, but the death of the slaughtered animals is certainly less painful than that by rabies, and often no other alternative is available. The procedure cannot be used with species whose numbers are naturally low or who are not able to repopulate their habitat rapidly, nor is it feasible in areas where rabies is enzootic at very low levels, such as much of the United States. The prospect of completely eradicating rabies from all animal populations does not look good, so the problem of protecting people from rabid animals is likely to remain for some time—and it is a not inconsiderable problem; in the United States alone, in 1975 an estimated 30,000 people were vaccinated because of bites from animals thought to be rabid.

When a person is bitten by an animal that may be rabid, speed of treatment is of the utmost importance. The best first aid is to wash the wound thoroughly with soap and water (or water alone if that is all that is available), thereby inactivating and removing virus particles before they enter the system. If at all possible, the attacking animal should be secured—not killed, unless it is so vicious that it cannot be captured without the risk that others will be bitten.

After delaying only for these matters, the victim should be taken at once to the nearest doctor's office or hospital emergency room. There the wound will be cleaned again, probably with a disinfectant such as benzalkonium chloride, and doused with antirabies *serum* or *gamma globulin*. Injection of serum or gamma globulin is also likely, and if it can be clearly determined that the attacking animal is rabid, a course of vaccinations may be begun at once (or 24 hours after administration of *immune serum* or immune globulin). Under some circumstances vaccination will not seem called for—if the skin has not been broken, for example, or if the bites are shallow ones through several layers of clothing, which would be expected to trap the virus particles. If the diagnosis of rabies in the attacking animal cannot be made positively, the animal must be kept under careful watch until signs of rabies do develop; this is the reason that the animal should not be killed unless it has to be. (Actually, new diagnostic procedures are quite likely to be capable of detecting rabies at an early stage, and the risk of killing the attacking animal prematurely is not as great as it used to be.) While waiting to confirm the diagnosis, the physician must make the difficult decision whether or not to begin vaccination. If the bites are severe, deep, and near the head, he may conclude that the danger of a rapidly developing infection is too great to permit delay, and proceed with the course of vaccination. This choice is especially likely now that new vaccines are available to replace the old ones, which caused considerable pain and carried the risk of serious side effects.

When the course of vaccinations is not given, or is begun too late, or is not successful—as is the case on extremely rare occasions—rabies may follow. Estimates vary of the percentage of those exposed but unprotected who actually develop the disease. One extensive study showed a rate of only 9 percent, but many careful accounts of those bitten by single animals suggest a figure closer to 50 percent. When the disease does appear, it is almost sure to kill the patient. Every year several hundred people die of rabies in various parts of the world. Occasionally a recovery is reported of someone who has been vaccinated (perhaps several days late) but comes down with the disease anyway. In truth, many of these cases may be instances of vaccine rabies, caused by the vaccine virus and less likely to be severe. Nevertheless, some very few recoveries may be genuine.

There is little that can be done in the way of treatment. Morphine is not given to relieve the pain because in many cases it aggravates the nervous excitement, but barbiturates may help. Dehydration, which results from the inability to swallow liquids, is treated by giving fluids intravenously. Breathing is aided as much as possible, and oxygen may be administered for this purpose. Intensive care is maintained. Such treatment makes the patient more comfortable, aids his body in its struggle with the virus, and increases the possibility that he will be one of the few who, almost miraculously, survive.

The first major change in method of preparation of the vaccine following Pasteur's work was the use of phenol to weaken the virus, rather than drying it in desiccators, which was inefficient when employed on a large scale. Beginning in 1919, a vaccine made up of viruses from rabbit brain tissue and *inactivated* by phenol at an elevated temperature (37° C) was much used. This so-called Semple vaccine (named after its developer), because of contamination with animal nerve tissue, suffered the serious disadvantage of occasionally causing attacks on the central nervous system, sometimes leading to paralysis and death. Better in this regard was a vaccine prepared from viruses grown in the brains of newborn mice (in which mature nervous system components were not present) and inactivated by ultraviolet light. But the most used vaccine since the late 1950s has been one in which the viruses are produced in duck eggs and inactivated with a chemical called beta-propiolactone. This duck-embryo vaccine is not entirely without side effects, but the severe neurological complications are much less frequent than with vaccines prepared from viruses grown in nerve tissue.

The chief side effect of the duck-embryo vaccine is painful allergic reactions at the immediate site of injection or over a somewhat wider area. On rare occasions vaccines experience anaphylaxis, a serious and sometimes fatal allergic response. To avoid foreign tissue components in the vaccine, the cause of these reactions, vaccine makers have now turned to viruses grown on human cells in *tissue culture*. In extensive tests, such vaccines have proved to be painless and to produce higher levels of *antibodies* than the duck-embryo vaccine. It is believed that 5 to 7 shots of the human-cell vaccines will do the same job as the 14 required duck-embryo vaccine injections. Already these vaccines are being marketed in some countries, and they promise to remove much of the pain and fear associated with rabies vaccination.

One innovation likely to result from the new vaccines is an increase in preexposure vaccination. Prophylactic use of rabies vaccine has never become as common as, say, smallpox vaccination because of the pain and side effects. This was the case even though fewer injections needed to be given to offer preexposure protection—only three were used with the duck-embryo vaccine. Vaccination has been limited to veterinarians, research workers, and others unusually likely to be exposed to the virus. With the new vaccines two relatively painless injections, with essentially no side effects, appear to offer full protection. As a result, it may now be advisable for all who risk being exposed, such as campers, to protect themselves in this way.

In 1977, experimental work on an oral vaccine for use in wildlife was halted when a scientist working with the vaccine unexpectedly came down with rabies, in spite of having earlier been given the duck-embryo vaccine. It was assumed he had been infected by inhaling the virus.

The antirabies serum or immune globulin that is given along with the vaccine, or sometimes in lieu of it, has usually been prepared in horses deliberately exposed to the virus, the serum being the cell-free blood itself and the globulin that fraction of the serum richest in antibodies. In either case the protection offered is temporary, a neutralization of the virus by already prepared antibodies. Unfortunately, horse serums and globulins contain foreign proteins and cause some of the same allergic reactions produced by the vaccines prepared in animal hosts other than man. Here again, help is at hand in the form of material of human origin. In this case it is antirabies serum or globulin from human hosts, usually prisoner volunteers who have undergone a course of vaccination and have high levels of antibodies in their blood. One such serum is currently being marketed in the United States.

Another class of substances is currently under investigation as a potential adjunct to vaccination—the so-called *interferon-inducers,* which stimulate the body cells to produce their own virus-fighting material, interferon. One such interferon-inducer, poly I:C, has proved highly effective in tests with both mice and rabbits in preventing rabies when used with vaccine. Unfortunately poly I:C is not a good interferon inducer in humans, and it may be some time before an effective one is developed.

Actually, there is some question about how rabies vaccines work when given after the person has already been bitten. Usually antibodies are rather slow in appearing after vaccination (or after a natural virus attack), and serve more to prevent reinfection than to halt an ongoing one. It has been suggested that the vaccine viruses block receptors on the nerve cells and prevent the *wild viruses* from entering them, without themselves going on to multiply in the cells. Another suggestion is that the vaccine stimulates the production of interferon and halts the infection in this way. The best guess is that the vaccines function at least in part by stimulating antibodies, which inactivate the wild virus, whose initial rate of progress in the body is unusually slow.

Diagnosis of rabies, especially in an attacking animal, is all-important in determining the risk a bitten person is under. A tentative diagnosis can often be made on the basis of the behavior of the animal, especially if an animal epidemic is known to be in progress. More certain diagnoses, of course, must depend on laboratory tests.

Dogs who have died of rabies, and less certainly other animals, almost always show the characteristic Negri bodies when slices or smears of tissue from the brain are appropriately stained and examined under the microscope. (The Negri bodies are especially likely to be present in the Ammon's horn area of the hippocampus.) If animals are killed prematurely, the Negri bodies are less certain to be found, and this is the main reason for preserving animals suspected of being rabid.

A newer test, one that is almost always positive in authentic cases of rabies and one that appears at an early stage (in fact, as soon as the disease is thought to be communicable), uses rabies antibodies that have been coupled to a substance causing them to fluoresce under ultraviolet light. The animal is killed, and a sample of brain tissue is treated with the fluorescent antibody. Where the virus is, the antibody sticks; and when the tissue is examined under the microscope in ultraviolet light, fluorescence reveals the presence of both.

The fluorescent-antibody test is rapid and accurate, and the most used diagnostic procedure for rabies virus today. But even when this test is positive, laboratories frequently confirm diagnoses by inoculating the brains of newborn mice with the suspect material and observing whether or not the animals develop rabies in the prescribed period of 9 to 14 days.

An experimental diagnostic procedure that can be applied to live animals depends on their having viruses in the cornea at the same time as these appear in the salivary glands. In this procedure, cells are taken from the intact corneal surface, treated with fluorescent antibody, and then examined as above. Although this test is desirable because it does not involve killing the animal presumed to be rabid, it is not considered as uniformly reliable as the test on brain material.

Now that the rabies virus is being grown in tissue culture for the preparation of vaccines, it is conveniently available for study. The individual virus particles have been observed with the electron microscope to be bullet- or thimble-shaped. They are relatively large (for viruses), about 200 nanometers long (roughly eight millionths of an inch) and 75 to 110 nanometers across. The *outer membrane* of the particle is covered with small spikes with knobs on the ends. Inside is the virus core, composed of 95 percent protein and 5 percent *RNA*. Electron micrographs show the virus particles forming within cells in the vicinity of cellular membranes and acquiring their own membranes from the cell as they "bud" off from it.

Because of its structure, the rabies virus is currently classed as a rhabdovirus ("rhabdo-" meaning rod-shaped), along with a virus of farm animals, the VESTICULAR STOMATITIS virus, and a number of plant and insect viruses. (In fact, most of these viruses seem not to be related to one another and to have little in common other than their shape.) The rabies virus apparently has few close relatives. Two African viruses, a Lagos bat virus and an Ibadan shrew virus, must be related because they look the same, cause similar disorders, and react with rabies virus antibodies to some extent. These viruses may, however, simply be local strains of rabies virus.

RED MEASLES. See MEASLES.

REGIONAL ENTERITIS, REGIONAL ILEITIS. See CROHN'S DIS-
EASE AND ULCERATIVE COLITIS.

REOVIRUS INFECTION. Reoviruses infect a great many animal species,
including man, but their connection with disease—especially human
disease—is somewhat obscure. The virus particles are usually detected in
the nose and throat or the intestinal tract (the combining form "reo" is
derived from the words "respiratory" and "enteric"). And the viruses
have been found in patients suffering from a variety of respiratory and
gastrointestinal disorders of varying severity, from colds to pneumonia,
from upset stomach to dysentery (see RESPIRATORY INFECTION and
GASTROENTERITIS). The virus has also been found in patients with
ENCEPHALITIS and HEPATITIS. But the evidence linking the virus to
the observed disease in each case is very shaky. This is especially so when
it is considered that reovirus particles are routinely found in perfectly
healthy individuals as well.

Recently, however, a virus described as a "reoviruslike agent" has
been discovered in repeated association with gastroenteritis in the winter
months in infants in a Washington hospital. Although the exact relationship of the new virus to the reovirus has not been established, the two
resemble each other physically, and the Washington virus may in fact be a
variety of reovirus.

The evidence linking this new virus to gastroenteritis is quite good:
some 50 percent of the infants brought to the Washington hospital with
this disorder in a November-June period were shown in various ways to
have intestinal tracts heavily infected with the virus, but only 8 percent of
children with other diseases were so infected. The investigators concluded that "the agent appears to be the major cause of diarrheal illness in
the young during the cooler months."

Since, overall, the association of reoviruses with known diseases is
problematical, diagnosis of reovirus infections must depend on identification of the virus and some kind of epidemiologic study demonstrating a
correlation of presence of the virus with the disease state, along with an
absence of other possible agents. (Ideally, the virus should also produce a
similar disorder in some convenient experimental animal.) In the Washington study viruses were detected in the stools by electron microscopy,
and signs of active infections were given by rises of *antibody* in the blood.
Although other viruses and bacteria were found in many patients, none in
as high a percentage as the reoviruslike agent.

Until more is known about the nature of reovirus infections, little can be done to develop systematic treatment or effective preventive measures. There is, of course, no vaccine.

Originally the reovirus was considered a variety of echo virus (see COXSACKIE OR ECHO VIRUS INFECTION), but the reovirus particles are about twice as large as those of most echo viruses and they cause somewhat different effects on cells in *tissue culture*. Three types of reovirus have been found, differing somewhat in the antibodies they cause to form. Reoviruses infect so many different animal species that they have been described as ubiquitous.

Reovirus particles are moderately large, about 60 to 75 nanometers in diameter (some three millionths of an inch). They are *icosahedral* in structure. The particles carry no *outer envelope,* but are said to have a double protein shell. They are unique among animal viruses in containing *RNA* that is double-stranded; furthermore, the RNA is in discrete segments, rather than a single piece as is usually the case.

RESPIRATORY INFECTION. Many viruses enter the body through the nose and throat and begin to multiply in the upper respiratory tract before they pass on into the bloodstream and cause infections concentrated in other areas of the body. Among such viruses are the POLIO and MEASLES viruses. Usually these viruses induce a degree of respiratory distress—coughing, sneezing, running nose—along with their other effects, but at times the other more prominent manifestations do not appear and the chief symptom is respiratory disturbance. There are also, however, a great many other viruses whose primary attack is on the respiratory system, and in fact virus respiratory infections, including THE COMMON COLD, are the most prevalent of all diseases. It should be remarked, also, that viruses are not the only cause of respiratory disease—bacteria, fungi, and other microorganisms can likewise do the job, producing such common ailments as "strep throat," pneumonia, and tuberculosis.

Confusingly, there are about as many different forms of viral respiratory infection as there are viruses that cause them, but there is little sure connection between the type of infection and the virus that causes it—that is, the same symptoms can be produced by several viruses, and the same virus can produce different symptoms in different individuals.

Proceeding in more or less descending order through the respiratory tract, we encounter the following types of respiratory distress: inflammation of the nose and throat, known as rhinitis and pharyngitis, respectively; inflammation of the tonsils, voice box, and windpipe, called tonsillitis, laryngitis, and tracheitis, respectively; inflammation of the major and minor branches off the trachea extending into the lungs, bronchitis and bronchiolitis; and finally, inflammation of the lungs, pneumonitis.

The common disease states associated with these various conditions are: colds, with runny nose and cough (rhinitis and pharyngitis); sore throat, with dry, burning throat and painful cough (pharyngitis, often accompanied by laryngitis and tonsillitis), croup, with harsh, wet cough and labored breathing (laryngitis, tracheitis, and sometimes bronchitis); bronchitis, with wheezing, rattling in the chest, and difficulty in breathing (bronchitis and bronchiolitis); INFLUENZA or grippe, with high fever, general distress, nasal irritation, sore throat, and cough (rhinitis and pharyngitis, sometimes bronchitis and pneumonitis); and pneumonia, with high fever, chest pain, deep cough bringing up brownish mucus, labored breathing (pneumonitis). Of these, influenza and pneumonia are the most serious and produce the majority of fatalities.

Of the many viruses that cause respiratory disease, the best known and those most definitely associated with particular disease states are the rhinoviruses and the influenza viruses (discussed fully under THE COMMON COLD and INFLUENZA, respectively). Although many viruses cause colds or coldlike disorders, most cases of the common cold are rhinovirus infections; and since rhinoviruses cause nothing but colds, it is quite right to think of them as the true cold viruses. And, again, although other viruses may produce influenzalike disorders, most cases of the "flu" are caused by true influenza viruses. The influenza viruses can also produce a mild, coldlike disease, but even mild "flu" is likely to be marked by fever and to be more debilitating than the ordinary cold.

Besides the rhinoviruses and influenza viruses, the viruses most often responsible for human respiratory disease are the adenoviruses, the parainfluenza viruses, the respiratory syncytial virus, the NEWCASTLE DISEASE virus, the coxsackie and echo viruses (see COXSACKIE OR ECHO VIRUS INFECTION), and reoviruses (see REOVIRUS INFECTION).

In infants and young children, adenoviruses typically produce pharyngitis and tracheitis, sometimes bronchitis and pneumonitis; occasionally such childhood infection is serious enough to be fatal. In adults, adenoviruses cause less serious infections, usually a rhinitis and pharyngitis that passes for a cold. In children's institutions and military camps the viruses are often responsible for epidemics of mild pharyngitis and conjunctivitis (inflammation of the membranes of the eye) or a more acute, influenzalike disease.

In children, the parainfluenza viruses commonly produce croup, sometimes bronchitis or bronchopneumonia. Usually croup is more severe than a cold and is accompanied by fever, but the fatality rate is low. About a third of the cases are thought to be caused by parainfluenza virus (almost all the other viruses mentioned can also be responsible), as are some 5 percent of children's respiratory infections overall. In adults parainfluenza virus infection is rarer and milder. Perhaps only 1 percent of adult respiratory disease is caused by this virus, and that tends to be chiefly a pharyngitis or rhinitis without fever.

The respiratory syncytial virus is the agent responsible for the most severe respiratory disease in children. Even when respiratory syncytial virus infection is limited to the upper respiratory tract, it is likely to be severe, producing a badly running nose and a heavy cough; fever is common. More likely the infection will produce some degree of bronchiolitis or pneumonia, and hospitalization is often required. Among hospitalized patients the fatality rate may reach 4 percent. In infants under the age of 6 months, this disease is a major cause of death. Yet, in adults, the respiratory syncytial virus produces only a mild coldlike disorder.

A virus that occasionally induces mild, coldlike respiratory disease in human beings is the Newcastle disease virus—normally an infective agent of domestic fowl. The other viruses most commonly associated with human respiratory diseases are the echo, coxsackie, and reoviruses. Most of the time these viruses are associated with other kinds of disorders, such as intestinal disorders or MEASLES-like fevers, but they have been isolated from patients suffering from respiratory infections that would otherwise pass for colds. Coxsackie viruses have sometimes been found with more severe respiratory diseases accompanied by fever.

Clearly, respiratory infections vary greatly in their effects. Some are undoubtedly so mild that the patient is only vaguely aware of not feeling well; others range from a mild cold to a severe, even fatal, influenza or pneumonia. The differences are in part related to the virus; some routinely cause more serious illness than others. Also, of course, some people are hit harder than others by the same virus. Generally infants and the old and infirm suffer the most, but this is not always the case—young adult males were the hardest hit in the great flu epidemic of 1918. Usually the deeper the infection penetrates into the respiratory tract, the more likely it is to be life-threatening. But again there are exceptions; for example, influenza can be fatal even when it does not lead to pneumonia.

Treatment of viral respiratory disease generally consists of trying to make the patient comfortable. Usually bed rest is advised. Aspirin is given to ease pain, lower fever (when that is present), and permit sleep.

Inhalation of steam is helpful, especially with croup. Hot liquids sometimes ease the throat, and cough syrups are frequently good. In severe
cases hospitalization is required. No drugs effective against the causative
viruses are in current use, though there are agents that have shown
activity against rhinoviruses in tests. Antibiotics are not used unless
secondary, bacterial infections appear. (Since ordinary pneumonia is a
bacterial infection, it does respond to antibiotics; viral pneumonia is
another matter.) Most authorities advise against using antibiotics in a
precautionary way to ward off bacterial infection, on the grounds that this
only encourages the growth of drug-resistant bacteria, which may be
more difficult to deal with.

Inactivated-virus vaccines have been developed for use against four of
the more common adenoviruses (out of some 30 known), mainly those
that cause *epidemics* among military recruits. In civilian populations the
disease is rare enough that widespread use of these vaccines does not
appear warranted. Since there are only four parainfluenza viruses and a
single respiratory syncytial virus, all of which cause rather severe disease
in children, it would seem that these viruses should be prime target for
vaccine development. No such vaccines have so far been developed,
however.

Most respiratory diseases are diagnosed in terms of their pattern of
symptoms only—that is, as croup, viral pneumonia, or whatever is
appropriate—because it is almost impossible to be sure of the responsible
virus unless that virus is identified in the laboratory. Since there is very
little specific treatment that can be used even if an exact diagnosis is
arrived at, the chief matter is usually to rule out bacterial infection, which
does respond favorably to antibiotic treatment. Bacteria, of course, can
be identified by microscopic examination of material from nose and
throat swabs.

For research and epidemiological purposes, however, it is often
advisable to identify an infecting virus, and then recourse is had to the
clinical laboratory. Viruses from nose or throat swabs are usually grown
in *tissue cultures* or fertile chicken eggs, in either of which they produce
characteristic effects. The usual *serologic tests* reveal the development of
antibodies in the blood during the course of the illness. Tests with known
antibodies or known viruses identify the particular virus, or its antibody,
found in the patient.

The viruses involved in respiratory infections are so different in
physical structure that it is quite clear no single structural feature can be
responsible for their common action in the human respiratory tract. The
rhinoviruses, like the echo and coxsackie viruses, are picorna viruses,

small, *RNA*-containing viruses about 30 nanometers in diameter (one millionth of an inch), with an *icosahedral* structure and no *outer envelope*. The influenza and parainfluenza viruses also are RNA viruses, but they are much larger and variable in size and shape, ranging from 100 to 250 nanometers in diameter. The particles contain a helical core within an outer envelope, which is studded with small projections. Finally, the adenoviruses are *DNA* viruses, moderately sized, about 70 nanometers in diameter, with a well-defined icosahedral structure bearing knoblike appendages at the vertices and carrying no outer envelope.

RESPIRATORY SYNCYTIAL VIRUS INFECTION. See RESPIRATORY INFECTION.

REYE'S SYNDROME. Named for an Australian physician who first reported the disorder in 1963, Reye's syndrome is a severe form of ENCEPHALITIS combined with liver disease (see HEPATITIS). It is of unknown origin but mostly hits children in the wake of virus infections of various kinds, chiefly CHICKEN POX and INFLUENZA. Influenza B is one of the most common initiators of Reye's syndrome. In 1974, following a nationwide epidemic of that disease, some 30 children developed the syndrome; in 1977, after a similar epidemic, more than 20 were hit. Death rates vary from outbreak to outbreak—40 to 50 percent is common, but in some epidemics rates as high as 85 percent have been reached. Various treatments are used, with somewhat uncertain success.

The patient may begin with fairly typical symptoms of virus disease, headache, sore throat, and fever. But soon he takes a sharp turn for the worse and experiences uncontrollable vomiting and bizarre behavioral changes, such as delirium, disorientation, and confusion—one child who insisted on dressing put her clothes on backward. Soon the victim falls into a coma and begins to undergo convulsions. Death may come while the patient is comatose; often it is caused by pneumonia, a frequent complication of the disease.

Although there is no real cure for Reye's syndrome, physicians employ a number of treatments with varying success. With encephalitis the chief problem is swelling of the brain due to inflammation, and this is combated with steroids. To reduce extreme pressure on the brain, surgery may be employed. Liver damage causes toxic materials to accumulate in the blood, and sugar and fluids may be given intravenously to dilute their effect. Exchange transfusion—complete replacement of the blood—has been used in some cases. Also used is peritoneal dialysis, the bathing of the intestines with fluid while still inside the intestinal cavity, a process that permits the toxic substances in the blood to flow out through the membrane surrounding the intestines, the peritoneum. For reasons that are not clear, these techniques work quite well with some patients, not at all with others.

Exactly what causes this disorder is not known. It is thought by some to be a secondary infection that follows an initial virus attack. More likely it is not a disease in itself but a condition that results when any of several viruses unexpectedly focuses its attack on the brain and the liver simultaneously.

RHEUMATIC DISEASE. See CONNECTIVE TISSUE DISEASE.

RHEUMATISM. See ARTHRITIS.

RHEUMATOID ARTHRITIS. See ARTHRITIS.

RHINOVIRUS INFECTION. See THE COMMON COLD.

RIFT VALLEY FEVER. Rift Valley Fever is a disease that affects mainly sheep, cattle, and goats, and only in Africa—it was first observed in the Rift Valley of Kenya. Occasionally shepherds and veterinarians are infected, and they experience a brief but high fever accompanied by headache, backache, joint aches and pains, and dizziness. Young lambs frequently die of the disease, largely from liver damage, and pregnant ewes often undergo abortion. In 1950 and 1951 a great *epidemic* of the disease occurred in South Africa, killing 100,000 sheep and cattle, and infecting 20,000 persons.

The virus is carried by mosquitoes and appears to be a typical arbovirus (see ARBOVIRUS DISEASE). A *live-virus vaccine* has found veterinary use, and a *killed-virus vaccine* has been developed for human employment.

RUBELLA. See GERMAN MEASLES.

RUBEOLA. See MEASLES.

RUSSIAN HEMORRHAGIC FEVER. See HEMORRHAGIC FEVER.

RUSSIAN SPRING-SUMMER ENCEPHALITIS. See TICK-BORNE ENCEPHALITIS.

ST. LOUIS ENCEPHALITIS. A group of very similar diseases, caused by closely related viruses, the St. Louis encephalitis complex consists of St. Louis encephalitis itself and the Japanese, Murray Valley (Australia), and Ilhéus (Brazil) encephalitises. All are serious, sometimes fatal, disorders characterized by signs of brain disturbance (see EN-CEPHALITIS), ranging from headache, drowsiness, and irritability to convulsions and coma. The virus that causes each disease normally infects wild birds; it is carried to man by mosquitoes. *Epidemics* occur chiefly in rainy summers when mosquitoes are plentiful.

St. Louis encephalitis proper has been characterized by one authority as "the most important mosquito-borne disease of the continental United States." It occurs in the far western, central, and southern United States, as well as the Caribbean Islands and South America. First reported in southern Illinois in 1932 and in St. Louis the following year, this disease has since been observed in epidemics from Florida to California. In 1975 an epidemic that began in Mississippi reached 20 states, with Illinois the hardest hit. In Illinois alone in that year there were more than 1,000 suspected cases and 65 deaths.

The Japanese encephalitis—known also as Japanese B encephalitis to distinguish it from another, quite different disease—was first described in Japan in 1924, though records suggest it goes back to at least 1871. It occurs in most of the Far East, including mainland China and India.

Murray Valley encephalitis, also known as Australian X disease, was first observed in 1917 in southeastern Australia in the river valley that gives it its more common name. It has subsequently been observed also in New Guinea.

Ilhéus virus was first detected in wild mosquitoes captured near Ilhéus on the Brazilian coast. It has since been found widely in South and Central America and the Caribbean Islands.

A notable characteristic of these diseases is the large number of *inapparent infections.* Mass testing for *antibodies* to the viruses in the blood of unaffected persons during epidemics shows that 100 or more become infected for every one that shows active symptoms of disease. Of those who do develop symptoms, many undergo only a brief, feverish illness, with a severe headache often the only sign of brain disorder. Such cases are the general rule with St. Louis and Ilhéus encephalitises, which are usually less severe than the related forms.

But a more severe encephalitis does appear in many patients—especially in those experiencing Japanese or Murray Valley encephalitis, though also in certain sufferers from the usually milder varieties. This may follow a day or two of the kind of mild illness described above. Often the encephalitis is accompanied by nausea and vomiting. At times, the whole complex of symptoms comes together. Usually, the encephalitis is marked by high fever, severe headache, stiffness of the neck, dizziness, drowsiness, mental confusion, lack of coordination, painful response to light, and speech disturbance. In children, convulsions are not uncommon. In severe cases of any age, coma begins early, and death occurs within 10 days. Otherwise, the fever generally lifts in 3 days to a week, and recovery may be quite rapid even in cases which have seemed severe. Complete recovery is the rule, but some patients are permanently impaired, showing mental retardation or partial paralysis.

St. Louis encephalitis hits elderly patients the hardest. They undergo severe symptoms, have higher death rates, convalesce more slowly, and are more likely to be left with some mental or physical problems. The older population in Florida has proved especially susceptible in epidemics there. The Japanese and Australian diseases, on the other hand, seem to hit hardest at children, infants being most vulnerable of all.

The viruses responsible for all four diseases have repeatedly been found in birds, in which they do not seem to cause illness. The St. Louis encephalitis virus has been detected in both wild and domestic birds—in year-round residents as well as migrants. Implicated are pigeons, robins, sparrows, ducks, and geese. Some rodents also carry the St. Louis virus, and they may play a part in maintaining it in nature between epidemics. The Murray Valley virus too seems to attack chiefly birds, but the Japanese variety, although it infects herons and egrets, has a preferred host in pigs. The Ilhéus virus also likes birds, but it is suspected of infecting monkeys as well.

All these viruses are carried by mosquitoes of various species of the genus Culex. (Ilhéus virus reportedly is carried by mosquitoes of other genera, too.) Most of these mosquitoes do not favor man as a host, though he is sometimes bitten, and the disease spreads to man only occasionally. It is reported that one of the chief species responsible for spreading St. Louis encephalitis, Culex pipiens, feeds on man only when temperatures reach 85°F, a fact that has obvious implications for the spread of the disease.

Depending on the mosquitoes involved, some of which are rural and some more urban, the disease outbreaks follow two patterns: the Japanese, Brazilian, and Australian diseases, as well as the St. Louis encephalitis in California, all are essentially rural, and field and forest workers are often the first exposed. But St. Louis encephalitis in the central and southeastern United States follows an urban–suburban pattern, with anyone likely to be attacked.

There is no really effective treatment for these diseases. Patients are simply made as comfortable as possible. Hospitalization is called for only when signs of encephalitis appear. Nor are there vaccines that would prevent them.

Hence, protection against these diseases can be accomplished only by mosquito control. Insecticides are effective, of course, but there are now many limitations on their use. One effective control method is elimination of mosquito breeding grounds, any areas of standing water on which the mosquito eggs can be laid. Rubbish that collects standing water is, for instance, a good breeding spot. Birdbaths are another. Many cases of encephalitis in Illinois in the epidemic of 1975 were reported to be near cemeteries, where the mosquitoes had bred in flower vases.

Individuals forced to work outdoors when epidemics are in progress are advised to use insect repellents. And since mosquitoes of some of the species involved feed in the early evening hours, people are often warned to avoid going into areas where they abound after dark.

Because there are so many varieties of encephalitis, diagnosis must be by identification of the causative virus. It is usually possible to isolate viruses from the central nervous system on postmortem examination, but it is very difficult to find them in the blood of live patients. Identification of the viruses, then, depends mainly on detection of rises in antibody levels as the disease proceeds. The exact nature of the antibody can be determined by *serologic tests* against samples of known viruses.

The viruses are typical arboviruses of the so-called B group (see ARBOVIRUS DISEASE). They are interrelated—with Ilhéus virus somewhat distinct from the other three—as indicated by the fact that antibodies to one react to some extent with the other viruses themselves. All are related to the West Nile virus, which causes a denguelike fever (see DENGUE) rather than an encephalitis. Yet, in spite of their similarities, these viruses are sufficiently unlike that they can be differentiated by tests with antibodies.

SANDFLY FEVER (PHLEBOTOMUS FEVER, THREE-DAY FEVER). A severe, but brief, feverish ailment, sandfly fever is of interest chiefly because it is the only known disease carried by the sandfly (Phlebotomus papatasii and other Phlebotomus species).

Attacks are generally of short duration—about three days—following an *incubation period* of three to six days. The symptoms resemble those of INFLUENZA or the early stages of DENGUE. There is usually a high fever (104°F). Also present are headache, severe pain around the eyes, and joint pain, but there is usually no rash. Sensitivity to light is common. The disease is never fatal and complications do not occur.

The disease is found in southern Italy, Sicily, Iran, Panama, and Brazil. In Europe man seems to be the only animal host of the virus, but in South America rodents also carry it. In either case, the virus is brought to man by the bite of the sandfly. Epidemics occur in hot, dry months, when the sandfly is prevalent. Insect eradication is the only way of controlling the disease.

In all, some 10 different strains of the chief causative agent, the phlebotomus fever virus, have been isolated in Europe and the Americas. In addition, two distinct strains of a separate virus, which also infects sandflies and causes sandfly fever in man, have been found in Panama and Brazil. This is the Changuinola virus, named for the river in Panama near which it was first found. Both kinds of sandfly fever virus are included in the general class of arboviruses (see ARBOVIRUS DISEASE).

SCLERODERMA. See CONNECTIVE TISSUE DISEASE.

SERUM HEPATITIS (SERUM JAUNDICE). See HEPATITIS.

SHAKING PALSY. See PARKINSON'S DISEASE.

SHINGLES (ZOSTER, HERPES ZOSTER). Primarily a disease of middle and old age, shingles is characterized by extreme pain in a limited area of the upper body or face and an outbreak of small pimply blisters in the same area. It is caused by the CHICKEN POX virus, which remains quiescent after a childhood infection and emerges years later, probably as a result of waning immunity.

Shingles has a very long medical history—much longer than chicken pox itself, which until recently was universally confused with SMALLPOX. Shingles was, in fact, well known to the ancient Greeks, who considered it and HERPES a single disease. In time the two came to be distinguished as simple herpes, herpes simplex, and herpes zoster ("zoster" from a Greek word for girdle, describing the pattern of blisters on the body). By the 18th century, chicken pox had been recognized as a separate disease from smallpox, and in the next century the possible connection between it and shingles was suspected.

Often shingles begins for no apparent reason, but it sometimes follows a few days after an emotional upset, severe illness, X-ray therapy, or treatment with certain drugs. The first symptom is a localized itching or burning, or an intense pain, usually on one side of the trunk or head, the limbs being rarely affected. The skin in the affected area becomes very sore and tender, and the patient is likely to be feverish and generally unwell. Within a day or two a rash appears in the vicinity of the pain, which quickly develops into raised sores, exactly like those of chicken pox. Scabs form rapidly and, within a week or two, drop off, leaving no scars. New crops of sores appear successively over the first few days in adjacent bands or rows (like house shingles, hence the name), with the result that sores in several stages of development are present together. Fever and general discomfort usually disappear when the rash begins, though pain and tenderness remain as long as the sores are present. In fact, in many patients, especially older ones, the pain and skin tenderness persist for many months after the sores are completely gone—an especially troublesome aspect of the disorder. In a very few individuals a full-blown attack of chicken pox follows the initial shingles symptoms.

Complications are rare, but sometimes motor nerves are affected, and temporary or permanent paralysis results. When the skin outbreak is in the vicinity of the eye, the cornea can become infected, with permanent scarring a possible result. Occasionally, too, the skin sores become infected with bacteria (as is true with primary chicken pox).

In most cases of shingles, no special treatment is necessary. Soothing lotions ease the skin and aspirin helps fight the pain. Antibiotics are used to fight secondary bacterial infections. Little can be done to treat the rare instances of shingles-caused paralysis, but pain-killing drugs generally give relief to sufferers from persistent postshingles pain. In extreme cases, nerves have had to be severed, but this is a serious step, not to be taken lightly, and patients are advised that even in the most recalcitrant cases the pain finally does subside. Recently considerable success has been reported in relieving postshingles pain with a battery-powered device that provides prolonged electrical stimulation of the affected nerve, but this device has not yet come into general use.

Probably the best news for all future sufferers from shingles is that the chicken pox virus is one of the few viruses that has been found to be susceptible to drugs. One antivirus drug, idoxuridine, is already being used successfully with shingles in the neighborhood of the eye to prevent corneal scarring. And two new, still experimental drugs, ribavirin and vidarabine, are currently being tested against shingles in the hope that they will lessen the severity of attacks and eliminate, or greatly reduce, the painful aftereffects.

Except for the appearance of the skin eruption, there is no resemblance between chicken pox and shingles, and for a long time it was supposed that the chicken pox and shingles viruses were separate, but possibly related, entities. Experimental studies of the respective virus particles revealed no differences, however (see CHICKEN POX for a description), and *antibodies* to one were found to be equally active against the other. Finally it was observed that susceptible children exposed to shingles patients develop typical cases of chicken pox, but no one exposed to a shingles patient ever catches that disorder.

Then it was thought that shingles might be the result of a fresh invasion of chicken pox virus in a person whose immunity from an early infection had begun to wane. But there is rarely any evidence of recent exposure to chicken pox in shingles patients, and often some trauma has occurred which might have served to activate a latent infection. For these reasons, and because of the obvious involvement of a nerve in shingles attacks, it is now believed that the chicken pox virus remains in the nervous system for years after the disease has cleared up, only to emerge again (as shingles) when the levels of circulating antibodies in the blood fall (and possibly when there is some outside stimulus to the nerve involved). Usually the antibody levels at this point are still high enough to prevent a generalized outbreak of chicken pox, but not invariably, thus accounting for the few cases when shingles is accompanied by chicken pox proper. In any case, the attack of shingles stimulates a new round of antibody production, and antibody levels then remain high enough so that second attacks of shingles are virtually unknown. (This is fortunate—most victims would agree that once in a lifetime is enough.)

SIDS. See SUDDEN INFANT DEATH SYNDROME.

SJOGREN'S SYNDROME. See CONNECTIVE TISSUE DISEASE.

SLE. See SYSTEMIC LUPUS ERYTHEMATOSUS.

SLOW VIRUS DISEASE. Most virus diseases are acute—that is, they come on abruptly and then rapidly progress to a climax, at which point they either prevail over their victim's defenses or give way before them. If the disease gives way, the patient not only recovers but is left with a degree of immunity to further attacks, either temporary or permanent, depending on the nature of the disease. But it is now gradually being recognized that some virus infections conspicuously violate this pattern; they are chronic—once contracted, they persist more or less indefinitely, often for the patient's remaining lifetime, waxing and waning, sometimes entering remission, sometimes flaring up with renewed vigor, but gradually progressing toward a serious outcome, generally a fatal one. Because most medical investigators have come to expect that virus diseases do not follow the chronic pattern, they have preferred to call such diseases "slow," rather than "chronic," but the meaning is much the same.

Actually, some ordinary virus infections do not quite follow the "acute" pattern. Thus, HERPES outbreaks, the familiar cold sores, flare up again and again at much the same site—and these flare-ups do not result from fresh attacks on the body by the virus, but from reemergence of the virus from a protected hiding place in the nerve cells. Also, the CHICKEN POX virus often remains in the body in some latent form, only to reappear in middle age and cause an attack of SHINGLES.

Now, however, it has begun to seem that other viruses too can remain in the body after the initial infection has subsided, and subsequently give rise to new infections, but these infections are of the chronic or "slow" variety. There is good evidence, for example, that the MEASLES virus acts in this way to cause the relatively obscure neurological disease SUBACUTE SCLEROSING PANENCEPHALITIS, and possibly the chronic PAGET'S DISEASE OF BONE. There is some suspicion that it may act similarly to cause MULTIPLE SCLEROSIS.

The GERMAN MEASLES virus is under suspicion as remaining in the body to produce ARTHRITIS, and perhaps DIABETES, although either MUMPS virus or certain coxsackie viruses (see COXSACKIE OR ECHO VIRUS INFECTION) seem more likely in this regard. The mumps virus too has been suggested as a possible cause of multiple sclerosis. Viruses related to certain animal cancer viruses have been listed as suspects for SYSTEMIC LUPUS ERYTHEMATOSUS and PROGRESSIVE MULTIFOCAL LEUKOENCEPHALOPATHY.

It is thought that PARKINSON'S DISEASE, too, may be caused by a virus, possibly the one responsible for encephalitis lethargica (see ENCEPHALITIS). There is some evidence that CROHN'S DISEASE AND ULCERATIVE COLITIS—both chronic diseases of the bowel—may result from virus infection. And, finally, it has even been suspected that degenerative cardiovascular changes—the kind that lead to heart attack and stroke—may be caused by a slow virus infection, though here the evidence is less good.

What all these diseases have in common, other than the "slow" aspect, is their "autoimmune" character—that is, that the body's defense mechanism is turned against the body's own tissues, producing inflammation, tissue destruction, and finally degeneration. It is assumed that the virus is in some way responsible for this process, perhaps operating in conjunction with an abnormality of the immunity system. Exactly what the virus does is not known, though it has been suggested that it enters certain cells and alters their surface to such an extent that the body no longer recognizes them as its own and mounts an attack on them, and possibly on unrelated, unaltered cells as well.

Not all slow virus diseases are autoimmune in nature, however; two rare and peculiar neurological diseases, KURU and CREUTZFELDT-JAKOB DISEASE, are not only not autoimmune but they seem to be caused by viruses that are so peculiar they hardly seem to be viruses at all.

In order to learn more about slow virus diseases, medical investigators have turned to the study of persistent virus infections in *tissue culture*. Normally when viruses invade cultured cells, they rapidly kill them off (as they kill off body cells when they invade them), but under certain circumstances the viruses and cells settle down into a state of uneasy toleration, with few virus particles actually being produced, though signs of their presence can be detected if great care is taken. (This situation is reminiscent of that with the slow virus diseases, in which it has been very difficult to obtain unequivocal evidence of virus infection, even though there are suggestive signs.)

So far investigators have linked such persistent infections with three different conditions: the presence of defective virus particles, the appearance of temperature-sensitive mutants, and the partial integration of viral genes into the cellular genes. Defective virus particles are small viruslike units that are missing one or more essential genes; they cannot multiply in the absence of intact virus particles. Often the defective particles suppress production of intact particles, and hence permit a state of persistent infection to become established.

Temperature-sensitive mutants are altered viruses that are unable to multiply at normal body temperature but do so at lower temperatures. Such mutants sometimes appear in cell cultures and, in time, drive out the more normal particles. When the mutants predominate, however, the cell destruction that would normally occur at body temperature is greatly decreased.

There is good evidence that virus genes* under some circumstances can be incorporated into the regular cellular genetic system, where they may operate to produce some virus materials, though not the intact virus

---

*Because many of the viruses contain genes of RNA, whereas the primary genetic material of the cells of the body is DNA, it might be thought that the two would be quite incompatible. Many of the RNA viruses, however, contain enzymes that prepare DNA equivalents of the virus RNA, and it is undoubtedly such equivalents that are inserted into the cellular DNA.

particles—unless all the virus genes have been incorporated, an unlikely event. Presumably such altered cells could produce the signs of disease themselves, or they could act as targets for the immune system, as suggested above.

At present there is only suggestive evidence linking any of these processes to human slow virus disease. But as more and more is understood about how such patterns develop in the test tube, the clearer their implications for human disease are likely to become.

Although the whole question of slow virus diseases is very much a puzzle at present, these diseases are of growing importance. Some—perhaps many—of the degenerative diseases of old age are of this type, and as more and more people survive the hazards of childhood and early adulthood, the more there will be to face these diseases. As the problems of the aged become ever more important for society, the slow virus diseases become of ever greater interest. (It has even been suggested that the major degenerative changes that occur with aging are themselves the result of slow virus infection.)

SMALLPOX (VARIOLA). One of the most savage and most easily communicable of virus diseases, smallpox is a bodywide infection marked by high fever and a characteristic red pustular eruption of the skin. Death rates are commonly high, reaching 40 percent or more in some outbreaks. Survivors are often pitifully scarred, and may be rendered blind or insane. Though the disease was once a major killer in much of the world, it has now been eliminated everywhere but Somalia, in East Africa.

Wherever smallpox occurs regularly, it is mainly a killer of children, but this is chiefly because older people have been left immune by earlier attacks. When the disease invades a new area, it hits all susceptible individuals equally, without regard to age.

Smallpox seems to have spread into Europe from Asia or Africa in the Middle Ages; at any rate, the name was coined in the 16th century to differentiate the disease from the "great" pox, or syphilis. By the 18th century it had become a major scourge, killing—according to some estimates—20 million people in Europe alone. It is said that 30 percent of all British children under the age of three died of the disease during this period. The Western Hemisphere suffered, too, as the European immigrants brought the disease with them. At one point colonial Boston saw 6,000 of its citizens die from an infection carried by a single sick merchant seaman. The American Indian proved even more susceptible: one estimate, perhaps exaggerated, is that more than 3 million Mexican natives were killed by smallpox following the coming of the Spanish.

Man's counterattack on smallpox began with the practice of variation—inoculation with smallpox matter to produce a mild case of the disease and, following it, immunity. The custom apparently originated in China, where smallpox is very ancient: and it was certainly practiced in Turkey in the early 18th century, for the wife of the British ambassador, Lady Mary Wortley Montagu, witnessed it there and had her own children inoculated. (She herself had suffered a nearly fatal attack of the disease, which considerably marred her great beauty.) An able writer and an influence at Court, she did much to promote the method when she returned to England. After the successful inoculation of two children of the Royal Family, the custom made great headway.

The attack of smallpox produced by variolation was usually light—probably because the virus was admitted to the body by an unnatural route, a scratch on the skin as opposed to inhalation—but not invariably so; deaths did occur. And worse, the smallpox caused by variolation was contagious—with the secondary cases fully virulent. Thus the practice was responsible for many *epidemics,* and although a few people were protected, many were sacrificed who might otherwise never have been exposed.

Both drawbacks to variolation, severity and communicability, were overcome by a new procedure developed in England in the late 18th century by Edward Jenner, an astute, well-trained, scientifically minded country doctor. Jenner had learned of an old wives' tale that dairy workers who had taken a disease of cattle called cowpox would thereafter be immune to smallpox. On May 14, 1796, after considerable preliminary investigation, he inoculated an eight-year-old boy named James Phipps with matter from a cowpox pustule on the hand of a milkmaid, Sarah Nelmes. The boy developed a single large sore on the site of the inoculation, and after eight days had a transient attack of fever followed by no further symptoms. On July 1, Jenner inoculated the lad with virulent smallpox matter—and found him immune.

At first, Jenner's method met with what today seems surprising opposition. Jenner had called cowpox by the Latin name "variolae vaccinae" (smallpox of the cow), and the word "vaccination" was soon coined satirically (signifying something like "en-cowing"). But the custom of vaccination grew, nonetheless, and in the early 19th century Jenner's "vaccine lymph," infectious cowpox matter, was distributed around the world. And as vaccination advanced, smallpox steadily retreated.

Yet, the battle was slow. Smallpox remained *endemic* in several parts of the world and continually reinvaded areas once smallpox-free. As late as 1920 about 100,000 cases a year still occurred in the United States. By 1950 the disease was virtually eliminated here, but worldwide incidence was still reported at 500,000. In the next 10 years this figure was reduced to about 100,000, but the number of actual cases is known to be so much greater than the number reported that estimates place the true number of cases at this time at between 10 and 15 million.

In 1967, with vast numbers of cases still reported from 44 countries, the World Health Organization undertook a courageous effort to eradicate the disease completely in 10 years' time. Although this task looked very difficult, it was not deemed impossible because, there being no animal reservoir for the virus, clearing it out of any human population means the end of the disease in that population—barring reimportation. If every area where the disease occurred could be attacked simultaneously, there would be no place left for the virus to come back from.

When the program began, smallpox was endemic in Brazil, Indonesia, Central and East Africa, and the Indian subcontinent, with scattered outbreaks elsewhere. As the mass vaccination program proceeded, the last cases were seen in Brazil in 1971 and Indonesia in 1972. By that year the disease in East Africa had been confined to a small area, but it remained rampant in northern India, Burma, Bangladesh, and Pakistan.

At this point health workers stumbled onto a new approach. Rather than simply moving from place to place vaccinating as many persons as possible, they would divide their time between searching for cases of the disease and vaccinating only those who could have been exposed. This "surveillance and containment" technique made it possible to clear the disease from vast areas by vaccinating as little as 6 percent of the population. (Mass vaccination needs to reach at least 80 percent to be effective.) With this new approach, Asia was almost miraculously cleared of smallpox by the end of 1976. (Countries are not officially declared free of smallpox unless two years of surveillance reveal no new cases—and Burma and Bangladesh, the last Asian countries where the disease occurred, were expected to reach that status in 1977.)

In Africa in 1976 smallpox had been limited to a handful of cases in Ethiopa, and WHO officials were hopeful of reaching their goal of eliminating the disease from the world by the end of that year. But soon reports began to come in of outbreaks in neighboring Somalia, and attention turned to that country. Here, too, the campaign seemed to be succeeding, and it looked as though the last cases would come in 1977. By 1979 or possibly 1980 the world should be officially and finally free of smallpox.

In countries in which vaccination has already eradicated smallpox, there is good reason to halt mass vaccinations because, effective as vaccination is, it is not completely innocuous—complications do arise, and in the United States alone some half-dozen deaths a year occurred when the procedure was compulsory. For this reason, vaccination is no longer required in the United States and many other countries. There is, of course, some danger in such areas that smallpox will be introduced from abroad, as long as the disease occurs anywhere. In 1972, in Yugoslavia, where no smallpox had been reported since 1930, 34 deaths resulted from a single imported case. The last known outbreak of the disease, in Somalia, seems to have come via a traveler from Ethiopia. In the United States and most other countries, a certificate of recent vaccination is still required of all travelers or immigrants from areas where the disease is found. But very soon this requirement too will probably be dropped. In fact, health officials have now begun to consider eliminating many laboratory stocks of the virus to ensure that they do not accidentally escape and start new outbreaks.

It has long been recognized that there are two forms of smallpox: the ordinary or virulent type, often called variola major, and a second, milder form, known alternately as variola minor and alastrim. It was the latter that occurred most frequently in western Eruope and the United States in the early decades of this century, but it is the virulent form that now exists in Africa.

In cases of variola major, symptoms first appear about 12 days after exposure. Usually they are a high fever, headache, bodily aches and pains, vomiting, and general prostration. Only rarely is a light rash found at this time. In some cases, especially severe ones, the disease develops so rapidly that the patient dies at this point, before the characteristic eruption occurs.

Generally, after three or four days the patient's temperature falls, he feels a little better, and the typical pocks begin to appear—on the face, arms, hands, body, legs, and feet, roughly in that order. At the same time a similar outbreak occurs on the mucous membranes of the throat and esophagus. The pocks start as reddish spots, but they soon become raised and filled with fluid. As these pustules develop and spread, there is often a second round of fever. In severe cases, the pustules run together until large areas of the body are completely covered, and the secondary fever is pronounced. It is at this pustular stage that the greatest loss of life occurs. Up to 70 percent of those on whom the pustules form a solid wall may die, and even among those on whom the eruption remains intermittent, the death rate is about 25 percent.

The crisis often occurs on the 14th or 15th day, and if the patient survives, the pustules then begin to dry up. Ultimately they form scabs, which drop off after 3 to 6 weeks, leaving brownish stains or scars. These frequently persist for the rest of the patients's life.

The course of alastrim is much like that of smallpox proper, except that every stage of the infection is less severe and mortality is low—usually less than one-half of one percent. The typical pustules do form, but they clear up rapidly and there is little secondary infection, a common complication of variola major. Alastrim, in fact, behaves in susceptible patients much as true smallpox does in partially immune ones.

Smallpox is thought to be transmitted by virus-laden dust particles or water droplets, which are inhaled and lodged in the upper respiratory tract. There they are taken up by wandering lymphatic cells and transported to the bloodstream. The chief site of multiplication is the blood-forming cells of the spleen and bone marrow. Ultimately, the large amounts of virus manufactured there are poured back into the blood, and this phase of massive *viremia* corresponds to the initial feverish attack.

Later the virus transfers itself to the skin and mucous membranes. As it leaves the bloodstream, the fever abates and the patient's condition improves. The visible sign of the subsequent multiplication of the virus in the skin is the pustular outbreak. The extensive damage to body cells caused at this stage results in the release of many toxic breakdown products, which are believed responsible for the second attack of fever and the severe reaction that accompanies it.

Because the patient does not release much virus to the environment during the 12-day *incubation period,* the risk of contagion at that time is small. Once the symptoms begin, however, that situation rapidly changes. As the virus multiplies in the throat, it is extruded copiously and the saliva becomes heavily contaminated. Viruses are expelled at this time into the air in droplets. The skin rash, on the other hand, does not become contagious until pustules form and the skin breaks, releasing virus-containing matter. Eventually the patient's bed linens and surroundings become heavily contaminated. Viruses may be preserved in infectious form in dusts in the sickroom for a year or more; crusts have proved infective after many years.

Smallpox is so extremely contagious that extraordinary control methods are called for. Every suspected case must be reported to health authorities immediately, the victim must be isolated, and all those who have had contact with him must be vaccinated (or revaccinated) and kept under surveillance. In smallpox areas, special hospitals are maintained;

otherwise, screened isolation wards are used, preferably air-conditioned ones with facilities for filtration of discharged air. All bedding and clothing from the patient is burned; tableware and other nonflammables are boiled or otherwise sterilized. Dead bodies are treated as fully infective, and evacuated quarters are exhaustively sterilized. Isolation requirements are more stringent than for any other disease.

There is no special treatment for smallpox. The illness is so debilitating that the patient is almost inevitably bedridden, and the best course is simply to try to make him as comfortable as possible. *Gamma globulin* is given in severe cases, but its effectiveness has not been demonstrated conclusively. Authorities agree that antibiotics do not affect the course of the disease itself, but that they do reduce or prevent secondary infection of the pocks; this may reduce fever in the latter stages and also minimize subsequent scarring.

In studies, a drug called methisazone has been given prophylactically with good effect to otherwise unprotected individuals who have been exposed, but the drug does not cure the disease once it is under way.

Thus the only really good control measure is still—after nearly 200 years—Jenner's method of vaccination, which is carried out much as he did it himself. For many years the standard method was to apply a drop of vaccine to the skin and then scratch or puncture the skin repeatedly under the drop. A jet "gun" for rapid mass inoculation was tested in the early days of the WHO campaign, but the best results were obtained with a special double-tipped needle, which holds a drop of vaccine between the tips. The procedure can be carried out without even washing the arm, and is so simple untrained workers can do it.

The reaction to smallpox vaccination in susceptible, previously unvaccinated individuals is as follows: a typical, small reddish sore appears on the third day after vaccination. By the eighth or ninth day this has become pustular and is surrounded by a large reddened area. For a brief period now the patient is feverish and may feel unwell. In another day or two the pustule begins to dry up; it then forms a scab, which is finally lost, leaving a permanent scar.

Individuals so vaccinated are considered safe from infection for at least five years. (Jenner mistakenly maintained that protection was lifelong.) Even with declining immunity, however, the vaccinated individual is partially protected and, if infected, experiences a milder case of the disease. Revaccination, which generally is routine and follows a speeded-up course, restores full immunity.

Some patients experience no response to vaccination at all or only a very brief one. The latter reaction may signify immunity, but the former is more likely to mean a failure of the vaccination to "take." Such people cannot be assumed to be protected.

Complications are rare except in vaccinees who suffer from eczema or who have impaired immunity systems. In either of these circumstances, a spreading, generalized infection occurs, which may prove fatal. Gamma globulin, occasionally methisazone, or, experimentally, a drug called idoxuridine is employed in such cases. An estimated one in 40,000 vaccinated individuals experiences a severe form of ENCEPHALITIS, with about 40 percent mortality. (Fortunately this complication almost never occurs in infants.) Again, gamma globulin is the usual treatment.

At first, following Jenner's lead, vaccine lymph was taken from cowpox sores on the udders of naturally infected cows or on the arms of freshly vaccinated patients. Since the end of the 19th century, however, vaccine has been prepared in the skins of live animals, usually calves or sheep, and such material is called calf-lymph vaccine regardless of the source. Calf-lymph vaccine is safe and seldom produces an allergic reaction. Experimental vaccines have been prepared in chicken eggs and in cells grown in tissue culture, but these have not replaced the traditional material. An innovation that greatly facilitated the WHO campaign was a freeze-dried preparation, which is more stable than the liquid type, especially in tropical climates, and can be made up as needed.

Correct diagnosis of smallpox is extremely important because the disease is so serious and so highly communicable. Even patients who do not themselves experience all the effects may pass the disease on in fully virulent form.

Diagnosis is usually made on the basis of symptoms alone, chiefly the skin eruption. CHICKEN POX, perhaps the most similar disease, can almost always be clearly differentiated from smallpox because the pocks are quite different. In mild cases of smallpox, especially in people who have been vaccinated, however, the pocks may be untypical or they may not appear. At the other extreme, victims of especially severe attacks may die before the eruption forms. In either case the physician must rely on laboratory tests to confirm the diagnosis.

If there is a skin eruption, viruses can be identified in matter from the pustules by examination with the ordinary light microscope (following proper staining) or, better, with the electron microscope. Smallpox viruses can also be shown to be present in pustular matter by testing against known *antibodies*. Characteristic pocks produced on membranes of fertile hens' eggs or on sheets of cells in *tissue culture* reveal the presence of the virus as well.

If pustules do not form, viruses can be detected in the blood by the same methods. In addition, a rise of blood levels of antibodies to the virus signals that an infection has occurred.

Most experimental work on the smallpox virus actually is carried out on vaccinia virus, the virus found in the vaccine. Surprisingly, this virus differs in some respects from both the smallpox virus and the cowpox virus that occur in nature today. There is, in fact, much confusion about the origin of the vaccinia virus. In the long period since Jenner's day, vaccine lymph has been passed back and forth a great many times between man and the cow (even other animals on occasion), and some strains of virus have been lost, with new ones introduced; it has certainly been many years since one was taken from a natural cowpox infection. The most likely explanation of the difference between the vaccinia and cowpox viruses is that the former is a slightly mutated form of the latter; but it is also possible that somewhere along the line smallpox virus contaminated some vaccine lymph and hybridized with the cowpox virus or simply mutated to produce vaccinia virus. One fact that must be kept in mind is that the reaction to vaccination today is exactly as Jenner described it—an unlikely circumstance if the virus has been modified in any major way. Because of this, the suggestion has been made that it is the cowpox virus that has changed, the old form being preserved only as vaccinia virus while a new one, perhaps derived from the smallpox virus, has taken its place.

Whatever their exact relationship, the vaccinia, variola, and cowpox viruses (and the virus of alastrim) look exactly the same in the electron microscope. Chemical studies, too, have shown no differences, though it is to be expected that detailed examination of particular components will reveal some minor variations. Also, antibodies to any one of these viruses are active against the other viruses. (It is this principle that makes vaccination with vaccinia virus effective against smallpox.)

Yet, there are differences among the viruses of the group, as is shown by the animals they are capable of infecting. In nature, of course, variola virus regularly attacks man and cowpox virus cattle, although the latter virus can spread to man as well. Other differences are found with laboratory animals. Thus, cowpox virus does not multiply when scratched into the skin of monkeys, but it does with rabbits. The reverse is true of variola virus; vaccinia infects in both cases. The easiest way of distinguishing these viruses in the laboratory, though, is by means of the appearance and timing of the pocks they cause on the membranes of chicken eggs. Vaccinia virus forms opaque white spots very quickly (within 48 hours), whereas variola virus (and alastrim virus) takes somewhat longer (up to 72 hours). The spots formed by cowpox virus are readily distinguishable because they have red centers. The alastrim virus can be told from the true smallpox virus because it ceases to give pocks on egg membranes at temperatures about 38°C.

The pox viruses are the largest of known viruses, the only ones visible in the light microscope (though just barely). The individual particles are roughly brick-shaped, with dimensions of 100 by 300 nanometers (about four by twelve millionths of an inch). As revealed by the electron microscope, they have an extremely complex structure, with a ropelike component wound into an intricate pattern just below an *outer membrane*. This gives the particle a somewhat beaded appearance, rather like that of a raspberry. Within this outer structure is a flattened inner core. The *nucleic acid,* which is presumably in this core, is DNA. Because they are so large (as virus particles go) and so complex, the pox virus particles pose formidable problems for detailed structural analysis.

SSPE. See SUBACUTE SCLEROSING PANENCEPHALITIS.

STILL'S DISEASE. See ARTHRITIS.

STOMACH FLU. See GASTROENTERITIS.

STROKE. See HEART DISEASE.

SUBACUTE SCLEROSING PANENCEPHALITIS (SSPE). A rare disease that hits only one person in a million, subacute sclerosing panencephalitis is notable because it is one of the few degenerative diseases definitely linked to a virus—in this case, the MEASLES virus. (This finding suggests that other, similar diseases, such as MULTIPLE SCLEROSIS, may also be caused by a virus, possibly the same virus.) The disease is a slow, progressive infection of the brain, with a fatal outcome in some 80 percent of the cases. It occurs chiefly among children and young adults and only among those who have had attacks of measles.

Evidence that the measles virus is responsible for SSPE is extensive. Studies with the electron microscope have shown measles viruslike particles in the brains of patients with the disease; specially prepared fluorescent *antibodies* to the measles virus react with diseased tissue; and finally the virus itself has been isolated from such tissue and injected into the brains of rhesus monkeys, producing symptoms of the disease. Epidemiological studies suggest that those who have had measles below the age of two are somewhat more likely to develop SSPE.

On autopsy, it is found that the disease, which is somewhere between acute and chronic (subacute), has caused a hardening (sclerosing) of the nerve fibers in many parts of the brain (panencephalitis). Symptoms of the disease begin—usually five to seven years after the initial attack of measles—with listlessness and inattention. Over a month or two the mental condition deteriorates, and in time spastic movements of the muscles are observed. Death generally occurs in a coma after about six months or a year of progressive deterioration. A few short-lived cases have been seen in which death takes place after several weeks, and cases of protracted infection, extending over many years, also have been described.

There is no cure for the disease, and authorities are not sure how the virus happens to enter the nervous system and produce the disease long after the original infection. One hypothesis is that a special type of measles virus is involved, with the property of remaining within cells and causing them to fuse with other cells, thereby spreading the virus. In this way the virus moves through the body in spite of the presence of antibodies. Most likely SSPE belongs in the category of SLOW VIRUS DISEASE, a kind of untypical virus infection, which is lingering and protracted rather than acute and short-lived.

At this time, no one knows exactly what effect the recently introduced measles vaccines will have on the incidence of SSPE (and any other such diseases the measles virus may cause). It can be hoped vaccination against measles will prevent SSPE by stopping the original measles virus attacks that in time give rise to it. But this assumes that the weakened or *attenuated virus* used in the vaccine is itself incapable of ultimately causing SSPE, something that only time and experience will tell.

SUDDEN INFANT DEATH SYNDROME (SIDS, CRIB DEATH).

The largest single cause of death in children between the ages of one month and one year is the so-called sudden infant death syndrome. This disorder is suspected whenever an apparently healthy child is found dead—often in his crib, hence the alternate name, "crib death" ("cot death" in Britain)—with no sign of overwhelming infection or other obvious cause of death. The unexplained loss is frequently an emotional shock to parents, who feel negligent or otherwise responsible. Authorities now believe, however, that such deaths result from a developmental failure of some sort, coupled with a minor throat infection, often caused by a virus.

In earlier periods deaths like this were attributed to smothering, either by the mother's body or by bedding, and it was not until the 1940s that investigators ruled out this possibility and concluded that the deaths are caused by disease or abnormality. Subsequent investigations have revealed that many of the affected children have a minor RESPIRATORY

INFECTION, such as echo, coxsackie, or adenovirus infection. Although such infections would themselves not have caused these deaths, they are suspected of being a complicating factor.

Investigators have also discovered now that many infants undergo brief periods in which breathing ceases—periods of apnea, to use the scientific term—and it is suspected that certain developmental abnormalities may be involved in such episodes. Possibly sudden infant deaths occur as a result of a prolonged period of such breathing failure. Often postmortem examination suggests that the infant has died in the course of a spasm of the larynx, the part of the throat that includes the vocal cords; whether or not such a spasm could be related to an episode of interrupted breathing is a matter of conjecture.

Authorities have suggested a number of possible underlying causes that might lead to sudden infant death, including an inborn enzyme deficiency or a neurological disability; dietary magnesium deficiencies and lead and cadmium poisoning have also been proposed. It seems generally agreed that any virus infection present serves only as a triggering agent, but the possibility of a more significant role for virus infection cannot be ruled out.

Statistics indicate that sudden infant death syndrome hits 2 or 3 of every 1,000 children born. In the United States this means about 10,000 deaths a year. A majority of the deaths in the third and fourth months are from this cause. Yet the disease is rare in newborns, and tapers off rapidly after six months. Premature infants and those of low birth weight are unusually susceptible. The incidence of the disorder is higher in large cities (possibly because of better reporting) and among lower economic groups, though children of all classes die in this way.

Until the cause is more precisely defined, there is nothing that can be done to prevent this disorder. But parents whose children succumb to it can already be assured that the death is not due to some action, or failure, on their part.

SUGAR DIABETES. See DIABETES.

SYSTEMIC LUPUS ERYTHEMATOSUS (SLE, LUPUS). Considered a rare and almost invariably fatal disease until very recently, systemic lupus erythematosus is now known to be not uncommon—some half million people around the world probably suffer from it (with 50,000 new victims added each year), and many of these are only mildly ill, though generally chronically so. A highly variable disease, lupus can have any of a number of symptoms ranging from skin rash and arthritic joints, to severe heart, kidney, lung, or brain disease. Technically it is classed as a CONNECTIVE TISSUE DISEASE, and it is most closely related to rheumatoid ARTHRITIS. Lupus hits four times as many women as men, and the typical victim is between 20 and 40, though the very young and the very old are not spared (the recorded ages of patients range from 2 years to 97). Although the cause of lupus erythematosus has not been definitely established, there is good evidence that a virus is somehow involved.

One of the more common early signs of lupus is a reddish "butterfly" rash on the cheeks and over the bridge of the nose. This has been thought to resemble the bite of a wolf, hence the word "lupus" (Latin for "wolf") in the name. ("Erythema" is a reddening of the skin.) Severe cases are likely to begin with high fever, arthritis, and pains in the chest and abdomen. ENCEPHALITIS, severe kidney damage, and heart failure account for most of the fatalities. In milder attacks, fatigue, headache, and a general sense of being unwell are often the only early signs. But there may also be anemia and a loss of appetite. The reddish skin rash and arthritis are perhaps the most standard features. A particularly mild form known as discoid lupus affects only the skin.

As a chronic disease, lupus is marked by distinct ups and downs. The initial flare-ups are often followed by apparently almost complete remissions. These ultimately give way to new attacks, however, of varying severity, and the general experience is that once the disease acquires a hold it never lets go completely—though at times years may pass with no apparent symptoms.

A characteristic of the damage caused by lupus is that wherever in the body that damage occurs it is always centered in the connective tissue, the supporting membranes, tendons, and ligaments of the various organs. Thus lupus damage to the kidneys, heart, lungs, and brain is associated with inflammation of the connective tissue of those organs. (Even the skin rash that usually characterizes lupus may result in part from blood vessel damage.)

Another characteristic of lupus is abnormalities in the blood-clotting mechanism, which lead to hemorrhagic effects of various kinds, including bleeding in the skin and in the various internal organs. Such abnormalities have been traced to the presence of *antibodies* to the materials involved in coagulation, but the source of such antibodies is unclear.

Treatment of lupus varies with the symptoms, but aspirin is commonly used to ease pain and fight inflammation. Steroids, such as cortisone and prednisone, also are used to fight inflammation—they are especially helpful during acute episodes. Antimalarial agents too are often useful, for reasons that are not clear, and some authorities employ anticancer drugs to treat lupus. In certain patients attacks are triggered by exposure to sunlight, and for them, of course, it is wise to avoid such exposure as much as possible.

Diagnosis of lupus erythematosus usually depends on clinical tests—the symptoms are so difficult to pin down that they are not of much help in diagnosis. Both blood tests and biopsies—often on kidney tissue—are used for diagnostic purposes. One characteristic of lupus is the presence of a unique kind of white cell (dubbed an L.E. cell) in the blood, tissues, and bone marrow; another is the appearance in the blood of so-called "antinuclear" antibodies—antibodies that form against cell nuclei and certain of their components. Recently, specially prepared fluorescent antibodies have come into use for the detection of antinuclear antibodies.

Like rheumatoid arthritis, lupus is considered to be an autoimmune disease, meaning one in which the body's immunity mechanism is directed against the body's own tissues. In arthritis, this attack is directed against the joints; in lupus, against many of the internal organs—most notably the kidney. Furthermore, most investigators involved with lupus believe that it is a kind of SLOW VIRUS DISEASE, a virus infection that develops in an unusually chronic and persistent fashion.

Although nobody yet knows for sure that a virus causes lupus, there are some signs that a virus related to certain CANCER viruses, the C-type picornaviruses, is the guilty party. (Not that lupus is a kind of cancer; merely that the virus thought to cause it may be related to the cancer viruses.) Although the evidence is still indirect that such viruses are involved in human lupus, a very similar disease that occurs in New Zealand black mice is quite clearly caused by C-type viruses.

In this regard it should be noted that scientists working with infected New Zealand black mice have had some success in treating them—on an experimental basis—with a substance drawn from certain cells involved in the immunity system, a substance known as soluble immune response suppressor. This material proved helpful in preventing the symptoms of lupus in mice, and the experiments raise hope that a therapy for human lupus could be developed along these lines.

There are many confusing aspects to lupus. Good evidence exists, for instance, that the disease is at least partly genetic, that a tendency toward it is inherited. This inherited tendency may involve the immunity mechanism—not only because it seems to take part in the disease process, but also because there are other signs that immunity is somehow partly faulty in patients susceptible to lupus.

THREE-DAY FEVER. See SANDFLY FEVER.

TICK-BORNE ENCEPHALITIS. Russian spring-summer encephalitis and two other disorders—Central European encephalitis and louping ill, a sheep disease that occurs in the British Isles—are often grouped together because they are caused by closely related viruses, lead to many of the same signs of brain inflammation (see ENCEPHALITIS), and are all spread by the bites of ticks. In the United States and Canada the Powassan virus, in Malaysia the Langat virus, and in Japan the Negishi virus are suspected of being minor causes of tick-borne encephalitis. These viruses are apparently related to the above three and may well be included in the same group.

Russian spring-summer encephalitis* is the most virulent of these diseases—the mortality rate is estimated at 20 to 30 percent—and it occurs widely across much of the eastern part of Russia. (In fact it is sometimes known as Russian Far Eastern encephalitis.) The *incubation period* is 8 to 14 days, after which symptoms generally come on abruptly—fever, headache, nausea, vomiting, stiff neck, and eye pain caused by light. Soon muscular weakness and drowsiness appear, and the patient may slip into a coma or undergo delirium or seizures. Paralysis is a serious sign. In some patients, symptoms continually worsen, and death results within a week. In others, symptoms begin to moderate after 5 to 8 days, and a prolonged convalescence begins, which may last many months. (In such patients a partial paralysis may remain.) Finally, some few patients show only the initial symptoms and develop essentially no signs of nervous system involvement.

Central European encephalitis, which is prevalent chiefly in Czechoslovakia, is milder than the Russian disease and often follows a dumbbell-shaped course, with two periods of illness separated by a few days of convalescence. The first period generally consists only of a mild, flu-like, feverish illness, which lasts for about a week. The second period, which does not always occur, consists of a sudden resurgence of fever, accompanied by severe headache, nausea, and vomiting. In a small number of patients, severe encephalitis or MENINGITIS develops at this point, and although there are few fatalities, permanent paralysis may

*Some authorities distinguish a so-called biphasic meningo-encephalitis, which prevails in the western portion of European Russia, whereas the spring-summer disease, according to them, is confined to east European Russia and Siberia. In its biphasic nature, this disease resembles Central European encephalitis, and may simply be a variant of it.

result. The disease has sometimes been taken for POLIO.

Louping ill, which causes a severe encephalitis in sheep, is rarely transmitted to man, though butchers, sheep farmers, and others coming in contact with sheep are sometimes infected, and laboratory workers handling the virus have sometimes picked up the disease. In human beings the disease runs a mild course, much like that of Central European encephalitis.

Both the Russian and Central European viruses make their home in wild rodents, from which ticks carry the disease to larger animals, including man. Among the animals frequently infected are goats, and it is well established that where the virus is prevalent, people can pick it up by drinking unpasteurized milk from infected goats. This is a most unusual mode of spread for a virus.

Small rodents, birds, and other animals carry the louping ill virus, which is passed on to sheep, again, by the bite of a tick. The encephalitis that the sheep undergo is marked by a peculiar loping or leaping gait, which gives the disease its name. Presumably people become infected chiefly by tick bite, although with butchers handling infected sheep carcasses the virus may enter the body through small cuts or breaks in the skin. With laboratory workers, inhalation of the virus has been suggested as a possibility. In any event, the virus is a negligible source of human disease.

The Powassan virus was first isolated from the body of a Canadian child who had suffered a fatal attack of encephalitis. It has since been detected in ticks, mice, squirrels, and groundhogs in both the United States and Canada, and surveys have found *antibodies* to the virus among a few persons in both countries. But no new cases of disease caused by the virus have been diagnosed.

Langat virus has frequently been detected in wild rodents and in ticks in Malaysia. Experimental infection of terminally ill cancer patients with the virus has produced encephalitis, indicating that human beings are susceptible to the virus, but there is no evidence that they are normally infected.

In 1948 in Japan two patients with fatal encephalitis were found to be infected with a new virus, which proved to be related to the Russian spring-summer virus; it was named the Negishi virus. This virus has not since reappeared.

As is the case with other viral encephalitises, there are no special treatments for these diseases. Hospitalization is required of patients showing the more severe signs.

Rodent control and tick eradication are the most suitable ways of dealing with the spread of the causative viruses. Where goat's milk is involved, of course, pasteurization is the answer. *Killed-virus vaccines* have been used in both Russia and Great Britain to protect human beings and, in the case of louping ill, sheep as well.

Exact diagnosis of these diseases on the basis of symptoms alone is almost impossible because there are so many similar encephalitises, though an encephalitis acquired by anyone working with sheep known to have louping ill may well be assumed to be that disease. A truly exact diagnosis can be achieved only by identification of the virus present. In fatal cases viruses can usually be found in the tissues of the central nervous system; in living patients viruses must be sought in the blood or the cerebrospinal fluid. In any such materials viruses are detected by their effects on cells of various kinds grown in *tissue culture*. Also, a rise of antibodies to the virus in the blood during the course of the infection will be shown by *serologic tests* run several weeks apart.

Although these viruses are all somewhat alike, as indicated by the fact that they cause overlapping antibody reactions, nonetheless they are sufficiently unlike that they can be differentiated by laboratory tests. As it turns out, the Powassan, Langat, and Negishi viruses are rather distinctly different from the other three, which are more alike. Also related to this whole group of viruses is the Omsk HEMORRHAGIC FEVER virus, also a tick-borne virus, but one which causes a rather different disease.

The virus particles may be described as typical of the so-called B group arboviruses (see ARBOVIRUS DISEASE). Not surprisingly, the viruses of Russian spring-summer encephalitis and Central European encephalitis are reported to be unusually stable in milk, and rather high temperatures are necessary to ensure their inactivation during pasteurization.

ULCERATIVE COLITIS. See CROHN'S DISEASE AND ULCERATIVE COLITIS.

VARICELLA. See CHICKEN POX.

VARIOLA. See SMALLPOX.

VEE. See EQUINE ENCEPHALITIS.

VENEZUELAN EQUINE ENCEPHALITIS. See EQUINE ENCEPHALITIS.

VERRUCAE. See WARTS.

VESTICULAR STOMATITIS. Like FOOT AND MOUTH DISEASE, which it much resembles, vesticular stomatitis is a disease of farm animals that only occasionally infects man. Most people who have contracted the disease have been laboratory workers who picked up the virus through cuts in the skin. But a few dairy farmers have acquired it from infected cattle, and detection of *antibodies* in many farm workers suggests that others have had *inapparent infections*.

In man the disease takes the form of a flu-like disease (see IN-FLUENZA) with headache, chills and fever, muscle aches and pains, sore throat, and fatigue. Symptoms generally last only two or three days, and recovery is complete.

Like foot and mouth disease, vesticular stomatitis hits cattle and pigs heavily, but it also affects horses and mules. Although the disease is rarely fatal to animals, the sores that form in the mouth and on the feet greatly interfere with normal feeding.

The particles of the vesticular stomatitis virus have a peculiar, all but unique, bullet shape, like a cylinder with one rounded and one flattened end. The virus seems to be naturally transmitted by insects, chiefly mosquitoes, as the arboviruses are (see ARBOVIRUS DISEASE), but because of the special structure of the particles, it is not generally considered an arbovirus. Instead it is classed, with a few other viruses, in a group called "rhabdoviruses" ("rhabdo-" meaning "rodlike").

WARTS (VERRUCAE, PAPILLOMAS, CONDYLOMAS). The relatively harmless outgrowths of the skin known as warts have, since the early 1920s, been known to be mildly contagious and to be caused by a virus. They occur on many different parts of the body and exhibit considerable variation in appearance, but the same virus causes them all.

Whereas people of any age are susceptible, older children seem especially so. In one study the age at which warts were most common was 15. Warts are spread by direct contact between individuals or by way of environmental surfaces. Infection is likely to occur in such places as gymnasiums, swimming pools, and barber and beauty shops. Genital warts can be spread venereally. Experimental transfer of warts from person to person has been achieved, and in this way incubation periods ranging from a month to a year have been determined. Although the growth of individual warts is limited, new ones do appear at nearby locations as the virus travels across the skin, especially along scratches or cuts.

Although they sometimes recur at the same or nearby sites, warts generally disappear spontaneously after a few months or years. Their disappearance is commonly thought to be subject to suggestion—that is, if the victim is convinced that the wart will go away, it promptly does so. But there is no documentation for this belief. Apparently, in such cases, the wart would have regressed anyway, regardless of the patient's mental state. Spontaneous remission is also the most likely reason for the presumed success of bizarre folk remedies and magic charms. Needless to say, the childhood belief that warts are contracted by handling toads is not true.

The most common type of wart, verruca vulgaris, is a rather large knobby growth found on the fingers and the back of the hand. Smaller, flat warts, found in groups on the hands or face, usually in children, are called plane or juvenile warts. Another flattened wart, the plantar wart, occurs on the palms of the hands and the soles of the feet—it is the only painful wart, and it may make walking difficult. Genital and anal warts, known as condylomas, occur in both men and women. They often become very large, presumably because of their warm, moist environment, and they are most unpleasant because of their location. Warts in the throat —laryngeal or tracheal papillomas—are especially troublesome in youngsters, in whom they may close the throat passages and necessitate periodic surgery. The so-called digitate warts are foldlike growths on the face and scalp; filiform warts are threadlike, and appear usually on the eyelids or the neck. Extracts of any of these forms can produce any of the others, depending on where and how they are applied to the body, a clear-cut demonstration that the same virus is responsible for all warts.

Medically warts are best removed by surgery, by freezing with dry ice or liquid nitrogen, or by burning with electricity or chemicals such as acetic acid. These methods may not always eliminate or inactivate the virus, however, and the wart may reappear. Plantar warts have been reported to be successfully treated with the drug bleomycin (which acts as a *nucleic acid* inhibitor). And recurrence of anal warts, said to be an increasing problem due to the increase of anal sex, has been greatly reduced with a vaccine prepared from wart tissues.

Because they are limited to the superficial layers of the skin, warts are the most truly localized of virus infections—there is no general discharge of viruses into the bloodstream, as occurs with most other virus diseases. In fact, it is difficult to locate virus particles in the lower layers of the growth, though they are often abundant in the dead cells that form the outer part.

It is important to recognize, however, that warts are a kind of tumor—the only human tumor, incidentally, that is definitely known to be caused by a virus. And the lower layers of cells in a wart do exhibit an increased tendency to multiply, though not to the same extent that the cells in a malignant tumor do. Whereas warts themselves are benign—that is, they do not invade the body and spread to new areas as malignant tumors do—nonetheless they occasionally do give rise to CANCER; and though individual warts are not themselves a matter of great concern, it is not considered wise to let them flourish indefinitely.

The warts virus—technically, the human papilloma virus—is related to the Shope papilloma virus, which causes warts in wild rabbits and cancer in domestic ones. Two other cancer-causing viruses, polyoma virus of the mouse and SV40, a virus of the monkey, also belong to the same group, as do a number of viruses that produce warts in dogs, horses, and goats.

The human papilloma virus is moderately sized—about 55 nanometers (two millionths of an inch) in diameter. The particles are *icosahedral* and have no *outer envelope*; the *nucleic acid* they contain is DNA. The viruses can be raised in *tissue cultures* of monkey kidney cells.

WEE. See EQUINE ENCEPHALITIS.

WEST NILE FEVER. See DENGUE.

WESTERN EQUINE ENCEPHALITIS. See EQUINE EN-CEPHALITIS.

YELLOW FEVER (YELLOW JACK). An acute, often fatal, virus disease of tropical and subtropical areas, yellow fever is characterized by high fever, the jaundice that gives it its name, and in severe cases the vomiting of dark blood (''black vomit''). The virus is carried from man to man by the mosquito, as was first shown by United States Army Major Walter Reed in Havana, Cuba, in 1900. Following this discovery, mosquito eradication programs virtually eliminated the disease from the large tropical and semitropical cities where it caused devastating *epidemics*. But a new pattern then emerged—one that persists today—in which man is only occasionally infected, still by mosquitoes, but now from monkeys and other jungle animals that harbor the virus. Fortunately several vaccines are available, both stemming from research carried out at the Rockefeller Institute in the 1930s by Max Theiler, winner of the 1951 Nobel Prize in Medicine for this work.

It has been suggested that yellow fever had its first home in Africa, but there is evidence of epidemics in Central America in pre-Columbian

times. Although the disease has existed at a low level in Africa throughout recorded history, there has never been anything there quite comparable to the devastating epidemics that swept Central and South America all
during the 17th, 18th, and 19th centuries. Some southern European cities
too were attacked during this period, as were those in the United States,
including some as far north as Boston. New Orleans was a favorite target;
the last onslaught there came in 1905. In the United States alone some
half million cases are estimated to have occurred in the 19th century.

It is all but impossible now to imagine the horror of these epidemics of
"yellow jack." They took a fearful toll of human life, decimating whole
cities and paralyzing trade and industry. The symptoms were particularly
repellent, and there was also the strange mystery of how the disease was
transmitted. It did seem clear that the disease was communicable—it
spread locally from block to block—but the connection between victims
was negligible or nonexistent. Physical contact itself did not appear to be
enough to spread the disease, though no one could be sure of this. The
sufferers seemed to be struck down almost at random, the victims more of
a vengeful deity than the working out of natural laws. So the discovery of
the *vector* of the disease was doubly welcome: it solved the mystery of
transmission and it pointed the way to prevention, by elimination of the
vector.

Actually, the idea that the mosquito was the culprit came not from
Walter Reed himself, but from a Cuban physician, Carlos Finlay. With
Finlay, however, the idea remained a hypothesis; Walter Reed and the
United States Army's Yellow Fever Commission, which he headed,
proved the hypothesis to be correct. They did so by human
experimentation—on themselves and others—with some loss of life. In
the course of their work one commissioner, James Carroll, proved that
the disease was caused by a virus; he showed that blood remained
infective after passing through a filter that would remove all bacteria.

It was left to United States Army Major William C. Gorgas to put the
findings of the Yellow Fever Commission to work, and in the year 1901
he scrubbed from Havana all trace of the guilty mosquito—species Aedes
aegypti—and yellow fever. Several years later he repeated this feat in
Panama, getting rid of malaria at the same time, and thereby clearing the
way for the building of the Panama Canal.

These and other early successes raised hopes that yellow fever soon
would be eradicated, would become "as completely extinct as the
dinosaurs," as Paul de Kruif wrote in 1926. But by 1928 it had already
become clear that outbreaks of yellow fever were continuing in Africa
and the Americas in spite of removal of A. aegypti. This led to
recognition of the "jungle" yellow fever cycle, in which monkeys, bush

babies, and tree sloths act as primary hosts for the virus, with the vector being not A. aegypti, itself essentially a city dweller, but other species of mosquito, which live in the jungle and feed on the jungle animals. Man in this cycle is but an accidental victim, infected under some special set of circumstances—as when a woodchopper brings down a tree and is bitten by the mosquitoes that normally spend their lives in its upper reaches. Once one human being is infected, of course, he may infect others, if A. aegypti is available, reinstituting the "urban" yellow fever cycle.

Today yellow fever is *endemic* in two areas: (1) a wide band extending across central Africa, and (2) most parts of Central America, northern South America, and the Caribbean Islands. Although the disease goes to the eastern edge of Africa, it has not moved across into India and Malaysia, where A. aegypti is abundant and the huge, unprotected populations would seem especially vulnerable.

There is no conceivable way of rooting yellow fever out of the vast, steaming jungles of Africa and South America. Elimination of the mosquito vectors is simply too big a job to consider, and vaccination or slaughter of the animal hosts would be, respectively, an impractical or an inhumane alternative. All that can be done is to vaccinate as many people as possible and keep the cities free of A. aegypti. Some large areas have been made completely clear of this pest, but as long as it is present anywhere in the world, the possibility of reinfestation is always a real one.

There is also the problem of preventing the spread of yellow fever to other areas, where A. aegypti abounds and conditions are apparently otherwise ripe for spread of the disease, such as Southeast Asia and the southern United States. Constant vigilance seems to be the only solution to this problem. Airport and seaport cities in endemic areas are kept free of A. aegypti, local populations are vaccinated and carefully watched, and all travelers to and from such areas are vaccinated.

Both vaccines in use today were made possible by Max Theiler's early discovery that yellow fever virus could be cultivated in the brains of white mice. A group of French virologists, using viruses that had become adapted to the mouse brain by successive growth cycles in infant mice, developed the first vaccine, known as the Dakar vaccine. (It was prepared from a virus strain isolated in Dakar, Senegal.) This vaccine, which is simply scratched into the skin, has been widely used in Africa since the 1940s. Experience there has been that the vaccine stimulates production of a high level of *antibodies*, hence offers good protection, and it reportedly leads to few side effects, though some 10 percent of the vaccinees develop a fever, headache, and backache. In other areas of the world, experience with the Dakar vaccine has not been so good: serious neurological complications, including ENCEPHALITIS, have been observed with some frequency.

To prevent such neurological difficulties, which are thought to be due to the virus's having been adapted to the mouse brain, Theiler began to grow the virus in *tissue culture*. After considerable time in tissue culture, the virus changed, yielding a new strain, which Theiler named 17D. This strain is the ancestor of the viruses used for most vaccines today—all, in fact, except those derived directly from the Dakar strain. The 17D vaccine was given to large numbers of United States servicemen during World War II, and it did a good job of protecting them from yellow fever; unfortunately, however, thousands of them subsequently developed HEPATITIS. In time this was traced to the human *serum* added to the vaccine to preserve the virus. The serum, clearly, had been contaminated with hepatis virus, and once the practice of adding serum was stopped, the hepatitis problem vanished. The vaccine is given by injection, or occasionally by scratch, in which case a much larger dose must be used. The reaction is generally mild, a slight fever on about the seventh day with, rarely, a headache and backache, as with the French vaccine. The 17D vaccine produces low levels of antibodies (compared to the Dakar vaccine), but protection is still good, and incidence of neurological complications is very low indeed. Both vaccines are manufactured from viruses grown in fertile chicken eggs.

The symptoms of yellow fever come on abruptly some three to six days after exposure. The first to appear are headache, fever, nausea, vomiting, eye irritation, back and joint aches, muscle pains, and malaise. In spite of the high fever, the pulse is unusually slow. During this phase, which lasts about three days, viruses can almost invariably be found in the blood. After this, the patient often experiences a slight remission, and then either goes on to recovery (in mild cases), or undergoes a new attack, with resurgence of the early symptoms, plus jaundice and signs of internal bleeding, especially the black vomit from stomach hemorrhages. Nosebleed, bleeding gums, uterine hemorrhage, and passage of black stools also may occur. In favorable cases the patient begins to recover after three or four days of this second round of attack. In fatal cases—which may include up to 40 percent of those who become clinically ill—there is usually evidence of brain involvement, with delirium and coma preceding death. Although hemorrhagic signs are evident in many body organs on autopsy, the chief damage is usually found in the liver, which is enlarged and shows extensive, sometimes almost complete, cell destruction. The early symptoms are those associated with *viremia*, whereas the later ones result from attack by the virus on certain target organs, such as the liver (leading to jaundice and hemorrhaging) and the brain (causing encephalitis and coma).

Complications are rare, and those who recover usually do so quickly and completely, though in some cases convalescence is prolonged. The severity of the disease varies greatly, depending on strains of the virus, resistance of the patient, and other, unknown factors. It has been suggested that blacks generally are less susceptible than whites. The presence in endemic areas of many people with antibodies to the virus and no recollection of having had the disease confirms that *inapparent infections* do occur.

There is no cure for yellow fever; treatment consists chiefly of complete rest in bed with careful nursing attention even in mild cases. The patient is not given solid food in severe cases but should receive plenty of liquid. If vomiting persists he may be fed intravenously. Analgesics ease the pain of headaches and backaches.

Diagnosis on the basis of symptoms alone is difficult in cases without jaundice or black vomit. In epidemics, of course, the suspicion of yellow fever comes more quickly to mind, and the disease is more easily diagnosed. Mild cases are most often confused with attacks of malaria, or DENGUE, hepatitis, and certain other virus diseases. In malaria patients the parasites, being of microscopic size, can quite readily be identified. But for certain differentiation of yellow fever from other virus diseases, laboratory diagnosis is necessary.

For laboratory identification, blood and tissue samples thought to contain the virus are tested against known antibodies in suckling mice. A sharp rise of antibodies to the virus in the blood, as determined by *serologic tests* against known viruses at intervals during infection, also identifies the invading virus. Some difficulty in laboratory diagnosis is caused by similarities between the yellow fever and dengue viruses, but the two can be told apart by careful tests.

The yellow fever virus is small (about 38 nanometers, two millionths of an inch, in diameter), spherical, and covered with an *outer membrane*. The particles, which are known to contain *RNA*, can be observed with the electron microscope within the cells after proper preparation. The virus is a member of the so-called B group of arboviruses (see ARBOVIRUS DISEASE), which includes the dengue and ST. LOUIS ENCEPHALITIS viruses, among others.

ZOSTER. See SHINGLES.

Glossary

antibody. Antibodies are the substances in the blood that detect materials foreign to the body (*antigens*) and, by reacting with them, neutralize them. Taken together with the cellular immunity system, the cells of which engulf and digest alien materials, antibodies are the chief defense against invading organisms. Chemically, the antibodies are complex protein molecules, the structure of which is becoming increasingly well known. They are produced by certain cells that are stimulated into activity by the presence of foreign materials, in a process that is not yet fully understood. When an infection is terminated, the blood levels of the corresponding antibodies and antibody-producing cells gradually fall, but a kind of memory of the invader remains, and a fresh appearance triggers an immediate, enhanced response. This memory and the heightened response are the chief reason that most viruses leave behind them an immunity, often lifelong, to further attack.

antigen. Anything that calls up the production of *antibodies* and reacts specifically with them is called an antigen. (The word, derived from the roots "anti-" and "-gen," might roughly be considered a contraction of the phrase "antibody generating.") Although the term could be applied to relatively large structures, such as viruses, it is more often used for portions of an intact structure or separated components of it. Most antigens consist of large molecules, mainly proteins, polysaccharides, and *nucleic acids*.

attenuated-virus vaccine. Attenuated- or live-virus vaccines contain viruses that have been weakened so that they no longer cause the full symptoms of disease produced by ordinary or *wild viruses.* (The term "live-virus" may be somewhat improper, as it assumes that viruses are in fact living organisms, a point on which there is no universal agreement.) The attenuation of viruses is generally achieved by growing the viruses for many generations in experimental animals or in *tissue cultures* until they become adapted to their new home (and maladapted to their old one). As a general rule, attenuated-virus vaccines offer better protection than do *inactivated-virus vaccines,* the other main category, because the live, attenuated viruses multiply in the body and stimulate the body's defenses much as a regular infection with wild viruses would. Also, a much smaller dose of the attenuated-virus vaccine need be given, thereby reducing the risk of untoward reaction to it by the body. Although there is, in principle, some danger that the vaccine viruses might mutate in the body to a more virulent form, in practice this has not proved to be a major problem.

congenital infection. A congenital infection is one that a child is born with, one that is acquired from the mother before or during birth. It is not a hereditary factor, like color-blindness, carried in the genes, but an actual infection caused by an infectious agent transmitted from the mother's body to the fetus across the placental barrier or to the newborn infant as it passes through the birth canal. Congenital infections acquired by the fetus early in its development are especially insidious in that they frequently interfere with the formation of organs and cause severe defects. Because congenital infections are acquired before the infant's defense mechanisms are fully functional, they are likely to be lingering and difficult to eradicate.

culture. See tissue culture.

DNA. See *nucleic acid.*

endemic. A disease is said to be endemic in a particular locality when it exists there on a more or less permanent basis. Often an endemic disease is maintained in a population at a relatively low level, only a few people being ill with it any one time. Under such circumstances, most adult natives are immune, having been exposed early in life, and the new cases appear among children and newcomers to the area.

epidemic. A disease is said to be epidemic when it is spreading rapidly, infecting ever increasing numbers of individuals. So-called epidemics, or disease outbreaks, tend to grow rapidly until they run out of steam as the susceptible population has become largely infected. Often, then, epidemic diseases exhibit wavelike properites, rising and falling over periods of months or years.

gamma globulin. A blood protein obtained by fractionation of the *serum* left after coagulation of the blood, gamma globulin contains the various *antibodies* produced in response to infection. ("Globulin" is the name for a class of proteins, and "gamma" simply designates the fraction isolated.) When gamma globulin collected from a number of individuals is given to a new person, it offers some protection against certain diseases, such as infectious hepatitis. The protection is short-lived, however, because the foreign proteins are soon degraded in the body.

helix. A helix is a spiral of uniform diameter and constant pitch, like a coiled spring or a spiral staircase. Many virus particles have an overall helical structure—that is, one in which the protein molecules that constitute the coat of the particle are arrayed in a helix around the *nucleic acid*. The resulting structure is cylindrical, somewhat resembling a cigarette.

icosahedron. An icosahedron is a 20-sided solid figure, each side of which is a triangle. Many viruses, including most animal viruses, such as the polio virus, are built on a icosahedral pattern, meaning that the protein molecules of the coat are arranged into an icosahedron surrounding the *nucleic acid*. Viewed rather crudely, the icosahedral virus particle resembles a sphere, because the separate faces are not easily distinguished.

immune globulin, immune serum. *Gamma globulin* or *serum* from the blood of a patient who is recovering from a disease, or who has recently been vaccinated against it, is particularly rich in *antibodies* against the agent of that disease (here, virus). Termed immune globulin or immune serum, such preparations are especially active against the disease in question and are often used in therapy.

inactivated-virus vaccine. A vaccine prepared from viruses that have been treated by chemical agents or radiation so that they are no longer capable of infecting cells is referred to as an inactivated- or killed-virus vaccine. (The term "killed" is somewhat inappropriate because it presumes that viruses normally are living organisms.) Inactivated-virus vaccines generally are considered to be less potent than *attenuated-virus vaccines* because the inactivated viruses do not multiply in the body and hence do not simulate a true infection. Nonetheless, the presence of the virus material does bring about the production of *antibodies*, and many inactivated-virus vaccines, including the Salk polio vaccine, have proved their effectiveness. The chief danger with such vaccines is the possibility that in the preparation some viruses will have escaped inactivation and will cause disease in those vaccinated. Thus, constant monitoring of the manufacture of such vaccines is necessary.

inapparent infection. Many virus infections are inapparent (subclinical, to use a more technical term) in that they produce no noticeable signs of infection. Such infections are nonetheless significant in that they (1) confer a degree of immunity on those infected and (2) permit the virus to pass on to others who may be seriously affected.

incubation period. Every virus disease—indeed, every infectious disease—is characterized by an incubation period in which no symptoms are observed. During this period, the infectious agent is finding its way into the body, locating suitable sites for multiplication, and then reproducing itself and extending its sway over the body. When this process has reached a certain point, the outward signs of infection appear. Typically, in virus diseases, incubation periods of a week to ten days are observed, although with a relatively superficial infection like the cold it may be only a matter of two to three days, and with the so-called slow virus diseases it may last for some months.

interferon, interferon-inducer. One of the body's chief defenses against viruses is interferon, a protective protein released by virus-infected cells and carried to fresh cells, where it acts to halt virus invasion. Each species of animal, including man, produces its own kinds of interferon, which is, however, effective against all kinds of invading viruses. It is believed that interferon is more effective at halting established infections, whereas *antibodies* and the cells of the immunity system ward off virus invaders when they reappear. Because of the effectiveness of interferon as a virus fighter, medical researchers have sought to harness it in the battle against virus diseases. But pure interferon of human origin is expensive and difficult to obtain, so researchers have turned to materials that artificially stimulate the body cells to produce more interferon. One such interferon-inducer, as this class of materials has come to be called, is a man-made substance, poly I:C, which imitates the *nucleic acid* component of the virus and triggers the interferon-producing mechanism. Although poly I:C is very active in animals, it has not proved to be a useful therapeutic agent for man. Nevertheless, it has aroused interest in interferon-inducers and raised hope that others will be found that will be useful.

killed-virus vaccine. See *inactivated-virus vaccine.*

live-virus vaccine. See *attenuated-virus vaccine.*

nucleic acid. The genetic substance of the virus, like that of all cellular organisms, is nucleic acid. Chemically, nucleic acids are substances the molecules of which are large, made up from many smaller units called nucleotides. The arrangement of nucleotides in the nucleic acids conveys information for the synthesis of protein molecules to carry out the functional activities of the cell or virus. Nucleic acids fall into two large classes, DNA (deoxyribonucleic acid) and RNA (ribonucleic acid), which differ mainly in the sugar molecule included in the nucleotides. In cells, DNA is the primary genetic material, whereas RNA acts only to help translate the genetic information into protein structures. In viruses, however, either DNA or RNA can be the genetic component, and the cellular mechanism is restructured to use this genetic material for the production of new virus particles. In the virus particle, the nucleic acid is protected within a protein coat, and it is released to become active only within a susceptible cell.

outer envelope, outer membrane. Surrounding the virus particles of many classes, most notably the myxoviruses—including the measles and mumps viruses—and the various pox viruses, is an outer envelope, or membrane, of mixed protein and fatty materials. Generally the envelope consists in large part of cellular substances picked up by the virus particle as it passes through the cell membrane on its way out of the cell. It is believed that the envelope is involved in the processes by which the virus recognizes new susceptible cells and contrives to enter them.

pandemic. An *epidemic* of worldwide proportions, especially one of some life-threatening disease, is often called a pandemic.

RNA. See *nucleic acid.*

serologic test. Serologic tests are blood tests designed to detect and identify *antibodies*—in this context, antibodies against viruses and viral *antigens*. Usually the tests, which depend on easily detectable reactions between the antibodies and standard viruses of known identity, fall into one of three categories: neutralization, complement fixation, and hemagglutination inhibition. Neutralization tests depend on the ability of the antibody to neutralize, or block, a property of the virus, such as inducing disease in newborn mice. Complement, which is a component of the immunity system, is "fixed," or used up, whenever antigens (here, viruses) and antibodies react; complement fixation is demonstrated by the failure of red blood cells to be destroyed by a special antibody. The ability to cause red cells to agglutinate, or stick together—hemagglutination—is a property of many viruses that can be prevented, or inhibited, by the presence of antibodies.

serum. That portion of the blood that remains after the blood has been allowed to clot and the clot has been removed is called the serum. This process takes out the blood cells and the various proteins that participate in forming the clot; what is left is soluble materials, most conspicuously the protein *antibodies.* Although ordinary blood serum is not rich enough in antibodies to be of much use in fighting disease, the antibodies can be concentrated by a fractionation process leading to the production of *gamma globulin.* Also, serum prepared from individuals recovering from disease, *immune serum,* may be rich in antibodies and so especially potent.

systemic infection. A systemic infection is one that is bodywide, not localized or limited to some particular body part or organ system. Although a few virus infections, like warts, are strictly localized, most—including even those such as mumps that appear to be limited to a particular area—are in fact systemic. What happens is that the virus enters the body, often through the upper respiratory tract, finds its way into the general circulation, and then, multiplying within certain blood cells, reaches essentially all parts of the body. At this point, specific tissues or organs prove most susceptible to the virus in question, creating the pattern of symptoms observed.

tissue culture. The raising of plant or animal cells in the laboratory, outside the organism itself, is called tissue culture, and tissue-cultured cells are often ideal hosts for viruses. Cultured animal or human cells may be used to detect and identify viruses, which cause characteristic patterns of destruction in the cells, and also to cultivate large amounts of virus for making vaccines.

vector. A vector is a living organism that carries a disease agent between susceptible hosts. With many viruses—by definition, with all the arthropod-borne viruses, or arboviruses—insects or other arthropods serve as vectors. The most common vectors of virus diseases are mosquitoes and ticks, which transport the viruses as they travel from host to host seeking blood meals. Some vectors are simply passive carriers of the virus and do not themselves become infected; in others, the virus does actually multiply, perhaps remaining with the vector as long as it lives. Certain vectors even pass viruses on to their offspring, which also become active carriers without ever having fed on an infected host.

viremia. Viremia—the presence of viruses in the blood—is a frequent concommitant of virus diseases. When it occurs, it is often a transient condition that occurs shortly after the virus invades the body but before it concentrates on particular target organs (like the salivary glands in mumps). Often the period of viremia corresponds with a state of generalized feverish illness, which may be the first phase of the disease process.

wild viruses. Ordinary infectious viruses, circulating in the general population, are often termed wild (sometimes ''street'') viruses, to distinguish them from vaccine viruses, the weakened viruses used in *attenuated-virus vaccines.* Typically, wild viruses are more virulent than vaccine viruses, which are specially bred to stimulate the body to produce *antibodies,* while not themselves causing the symptoms of disease.

Bibliography

～～～

For the general reader, there is not much available on virus diseases. To be sure, many of them are mentioned or discussed in home medical dictionaries and encyclopedias, but the entries are likely to be brief and not go beyond the what-to-do-when-Johnny-has-a-cold stage. A detailed general account of virus diseases, however, is contained in my *Viruses: The Smallest Enemy* (New York: Crown, 1974).

As source materials for this book, I have regularly consulted a great many reference works, among them the following:

KRUGMAN, SAUL, and ROBERT WARD. *Infectious Diseases of Children*. 4th ed. St. Louis: C. V. Mosby, 1968. A standard guide to childhood diseases for the medical practitioner.

RHODES, A. J., and C. E. VAN ROOYEN. *Textbook of Virology*. 5th ed. Baltimore: Williams and Wilkins, 1968. A very complete sourcebook "for students and practitioners of medicine and the other health sciences."

RIVERS, THOMAS M. *Viral and Rickettsial Infections of Man*. 1st ed. Philadelphia: Lippincott, 1948. The first great classic text in medical virology. Contains much still of value. The current (4th) edition is edited by Frank L. Horsfall and Igor Tamm (Philadelphia: Lippincott, 1965).

SINGER, CHARLES, and E. A. UNDERWOOD. *A Short History of Medicine*. 2nd ed. New York: Oxford University Press, 1962. A concise but detailed guide to medical history.

In addition, to verify detailed bits of information, I have turned
repeatedly to the redoubtable *Encyclopaedia Britannica* and to medical
dictionaries and encyclopedias too numerous to mention.

For current information I have relied heavily on newspapers, popular
magazines, *Science, Scientific American,* and such general medical
publications as *Medical Tribune, Medical World News,* and the *Journal
of the American Medical Association.* Often such reference material
supports little more than a word or two in this book, and I have not
attempted to document these sources in detail. A classified listing of a few
of the significant sources follows:

Antivirus drugs

BURKE, DEREK C. "The Status of Interferon." *Scientific American* 236
(4):42 (April 1977).

KILHAM, LAWRENCE, and V. H. FERM. "Congenital Anomalies Induced in
Hamster Embryos with Ribavirin." *Science* 195:413 (January 28, 1977).

MAUGH, THOMAS H., II. "Chemotherapy: Antiviral Agents Come of Age."
Science 192:128 (April 9, 1976).

Arthritis

Arthritis: The Basic Facts. The Arthritis Foundation, 1976.

JAYSON, M. I. V., and A. ST. J. DIXON. *Understanding Arthritis and
Rheumatism.* New York: Random House, 1974.

SOKOLOFF, LEON. *The Biology of Degenerative Joint Disease.* Chicago:
University of Chicago Press, 1969.

STEERE, ALLEN C., *et al.* "Erythema Chronicum Migrans and Lyme
Arthritis: Cryoimmunoglobulins and Clinical Activity of Skin and
Joints." *Science* 196:1121 (June 3, 1977).

Cancer

Cancer Questions and Answers about Rates and Risks. DHEW Pub. #(NIH)
76-1040. U.S. Department of Health, Education and Welfare, revised
1975.

GALLAGHER, ROBERT E., and ROBERT C. GALLO. "Type C RNA Tumor
Virus Isolated from Cultured Human Acute Myelogenous Leukemia
Cells." *Science* 187:350 (January 31, 1975).

*Listen to Your Body: Seven Signals That Can Save Your Life. . . If You See
Your Doctor!* American Cancer Society, n.d.

MARX, JEAN L. "Breast Cancer Research: Problems and Progress." *Science*
184:1162 (June 14, 1974).

MAUGH, THOMAS H., II. "Leukemia: Much Is Known, But the Picture Is
Still Confused." *Science* 185:48 (July 5, 1974).

———. "Leukemia: A Second Human Tumor Virus." *Science* 187:335
(January 31, 1975).

RAPP, FRED, and DIANA WESTMORELAND. "Do Viruses Cause Cancer in Man?" *Ca: A Cancer Journal for Clinicians.* 25(4):215 (July/August 1975).

The common cold
DYKES, M. H. M., and P. MEIER. "Ascorbic Acid and the Common Cold." *Journal of the American Medical Association* 231(10):1073 (March 10, 1975).

PAULING, LINUS. *Vitamin C and the Common Cold.* San Francisco: W. H. Freeman, 1970.

Creutzfeldt-Jakob disease
ALTER, MILTON, and ESTHER KAHANA. "Creutzfeldt-Jakob Disease among Libyan Jews in Israel." *Science* 192:428 (April 30, 1976).

HERZBERG, L., *et al.* "Creutzfeldt-Jakob Disease: Hypothesis for High Incidence in Libyan Jews in Israel." *Science* 186:848 (November 29, 1974).

KAHANA, ESTHER, *et al.* "Creutzfeldt-Jakob Disease: Focus among Libyan Jews in Israel." *Science* 183:90 (January 11, 1974).

MANUELIDIS, ELIAS E. "Transmission of Creutzfeldt-Jakob Disease from Man to the Guinea Pig." *Science* 190:571 (November 7, 1975).

Crohn's disease and ulcerative colitis
CAVE, DAVID R. "Crohn's Disease and Ulcerative Colitis." *INFLO* 9(4):1 (Winter 1977).

Cytomegalovirus infection
GEDER, LASZLO, *et al.* "Oncogenic Transformation of Human Embryo Lung Cells by Human Cytomegalovirus." *Science* 192:1134 (June 11, 1976).

KRECH, U. H., *et al. Cytomegalovirus Infections of Man.* New York: S. Karger, 1971.

MARX, JEAN L. "Cytomegalovirus: A Major Cause of Birth Defects." *Science* 190:1184 (December 19, 1975).

Dengue
HOTTA, SUSUMU. *Dengue and Related Hemorrhagic Diseases.* St. Louis: Warren H. Green, 1969.

Diabetes
MAUGH, THOMAS H., II. "Diabetes: Epidemiology Suggests a Viral Connection." *Science* 188:347 (April 25, 1975).

————. "Diabetes (II): Model Systems Indicate Viruses a Cause." *Science* 188:436 (May 2, 1975).

Gastroenteritis

KAPIKIAN, ALBERT Z., et al. "Vizualization by Immune Electron Microscopy of a 27 nm. Particle Associated with Acute Infectious Nonbacterial Gastroenteritis." *Journal of Virology* 10(5):1075 (1972).

————. "Human Reovirus-like Agent as the Major Pathogen Associated with 'Winter' Gastroenteritis in Hospitalized Infants and Young Children." *New England Journal of Medicine* 294(18):965 (April 29, 1976).

————. "Reovirus-like Agent in Stools: Association with Infantile Diarrhea and Development of Serologic Tests." *Science* 185:1049 (September 20, 1974).

German measles

COOPER, LOUIS Z. "German Measles." *Scientific American* 215(1):30 (July 1966).

MODLIN, JOHN F., et al. "Risk of Congenital Abnormality after Inadvertent Rubella Vaccination of Pregnant Women." *New England Journal of Medicine* 294(18):972 (April 29, 1976).

Guillain-Barré syndrome

BOFFEY, PHILIP M. "Guillain-Barré: Rare Disease Paralyzes Swine Flu Campaign." *Science* 195:155 (January 14, 1977).

Hemorrhagic fever

SMORODINTSEV, A. A., et al. *Hemorrhagic Fevers.* Translated from Russian. Jerusalem: Israel Prog am for Scientific Translations, 1964. (Available from Office of Technical Services, U.S. Department of Commerce.)

Hepatitis

BLUMBERG, BARUCH S. "Australia Antigen and the Biology of Hepatitis B." *Science* 197:17 (July 1, 1977).

FEINSTONE, S. M., et al. "Hepatitis A: Detection by Immune Electron Microscopy of a Viruslike Antigen Associated with Acute Illness." *Science* 182:1026 (December 7, 1973).

MAHONEY, PAUL, et al. "Australia Antigen: Detection and Transmission in Shellfish." *Science* 183:80 (January 11, 1974).

MAUGH, THOMAS H., II. "Hepatitis B: A New Vaccine Ready for Human Testing." *Science* 188:137 (April 11, 1975).

MELNICK, JOSEPH L., et al. "Viral Hepatitis." *Scientific American* 237(1):44 (July 1977).

ZUCKERMAN, A. J., and C. R. HOWARD. "Hepatitis B Vaccine: Tests in Humans." *Science* 191:1126 (March 19, 1976).

Herpes

PRICE, RICHARD W., et al. "Latent Infection of Sensory Ganglia with

Herpes Simplex Virus: Efficacy of Immunization. *Science* 188:938 (May 30, 1975).

WALZ, M. ANTOINETTE, *et al.* "Latent Ganglionic Infection with Herpes Simplex Virus Types 1 and 2: Viral Reactivation in Vivo after Neurectomy." *Science* 184:1185 (June 14, 1974).

Influenza

BOFFEY, PHILIP M. "Anatomy of a Decision: How the Nation Declared War on Swine Flu." *Science* 192:636 (May 14, 1976).

————. "Swine Flu Vaccination Campaign: The Scientific Controversy Mounts." *Science* 193:559 (August 13, 1976).

————. "Swine Flu Vaccine: A Component Is Missing." *Science* 193:1224 (September 24, 1976).

————. "Swine Flu: Were the Three Deaths in Pittsburgh a Coincidence?" *Science* 194:590 (November 5, 1976).

PALESE, PETER, *et al.* "Genetic Composition of a High-Yielding Influenza A Virus Recombinant: A Vaccine Strain Against 'Swine' Influenza." *Science* 194:334 (October 15, 1976).

Lassa fever

FULLER, JOHN G. *Fever!* [A novel.] New York: Dutton, 1974.

MONATH, THOMAS P., *et al.* "Lassa Virus Isolation from *Mastomys natalensis* Rodents during an Epidemic in Sierra Leone." *Science* 185:263 (July 19, 1974).

Lymphocytic choriomeningitis

HOTCHIN, JOHN, *et al.* "Lymphocytic Choriomeningitis in a Hamster Colony Causes Infection of Hospital Personnel." *Science* 185:1173 (September 27, 1974).

Multiple sclerosis

MAUGH, THOMAS H., II. "Multiple Sclerosis: Genetic Link, Viruses Suspected." *Science* 195:667 (February 18, 1977).

————. "Multiple Sclerosis: Two or More Viruses May be Involved." *Science* 195:768 (February 25, 1977).

————. "The EAE Model: A Tentative Connection to Multiple Sclerosis." *Science* 195:969 (March 11, 1977).

Paget's disease of bone

MILLS, BARBARA G., and FREDERICK R. SINGER. "Nuclear Inclusions in Paget's Disease of Bone." *Science* 194:20 (October 8, 1976).

Polio

BOFFEY, PHILIP M. "Polio: Salk Challenges Safety of Sabin's Live Virus Vaccine." *Science* 196:35 (April 1, 1977).

SALK, JONAS, and DARRELL SALK. "Control of Influenza and Poliomyelitis with Killed Virus Vaccines." *Science* 195:834 (March 4, 1977).

Rabies
FELDMANN, BRUCE M. "Rabies Shots." *Science* 183:1248 (March 29, 1974).
NAGANO, YASUITE, and FRED M. DAVENPORT. *Rabies*. Baltimore: University Park Press, 1971.
REGAMEY, R. H., *et al.*, eds. *International Symposium on Rabies (II)*. Basel: S. Karger, 1974.
WEST, GEOFFREY P. *Rabies in Animal and Man*. New York: Arco, 1973.

Slow virus diseases
MARX, JEAN L. "Persistent Infections: The Role of Viruses." *Science* 196:151 (April 8, 1977).

Smallpox
BOFFEY, PHILIP M. "Smallpox: Outbreak in Somalia Slows Rapid Progress toward Eradication." *Science* 196:1298 (June 17, 1977).
HENDERSON, DONALD A. "The Eradication of Smallpox." *Scientific American* 235(4):25 (October 1976).

Subacute sclerosing panencephalitis
ALBRECHT, PAUL, *et al.* "Subacute Sclerosing Panencephalitis: Experimental Infection in Primates." *Science* 195:64 (January 7, 1977).

Sudden infant death syndrome
BECKWITH, J. BRUCE. *The Sudden Infant Death Syndrome*. DHEW Publication #(HSA)75-5137. U.S. Department of Health, Education and Welfare, 1975.
MARX, JEAN L. "Crib Death: Some Promising Leads But No Solution Yet." *Science* 189:367 (August 1, 1975).
NAEYE, RICHARD L. "Hypoxemia and the Sudden Infant Death Syndrome." *Science* 186:837 (November 29, 1974).
NAEYE, RICHARD L., *et al.* "Carotid Body in the Sudden Infant Death Syndrome." *Science* 191:567 (February 13, 1976).
SHANNON, D. C., and D. KELLY. "Impaired Regulation of Alveolar Ventilation and the Sudden Infant Death Syndrome." *Science* 197:367 (July 22, 1977).

Systemic lupus erythematosus
KRAKAUER, R. S., *et al.* "Prevention of Autoimmunity in Experimental Lupus Erythematosus by Soluble Immune Response Suppressor." *Science* 196:56 (April 1, 1977).

MARX, JEAN L. "Autoimmune Disease: New Evidence About Lupus."
  Science 192:1089 (June 11, 1976).
MIOTTI, ANGELICA B. "Hemostatic Function Disorders in SLE." *INFLO*
  9(2):1 (Summer 1976).
SLE: Systemic Lupus Erythematosus. The Arthritis Foundation, n.d.
TOURVILLE, DONALD R. "Immunofluorescence in Diagnosing SLE."
  INFLO 9(2):1 (Summer 1976).

Index

Locations of main entries are indicated by page numbers in boldface type. The selection of index entries needs little explanation, except that symptoms which help discriminate diseases are listed, whereas those that apply to virtually all virus diseases, such as headache and fever, are not, except under special circumstances.